Surgical Management of Paraesophageal Hernia

Editors

INDERPAL S. SARKARIA
ABBAS EL-SAYED ABBAS

THORACIC SURGERY CLINICS

www.thoracic.theclinics.com

Consulting Editor
M. BLAIR MARSHALL

November 2019 • Volume 29 • Number 4

ELSEVIER

1600 John F. Kennedy Boulevard • Suite 1800 • Philadelphia, Pennsylvania, 19103-2899

http://www.thoracic.theclinics.com

THORACIC SURGERY CLINICS Volume 29, Number 4
November 2019 ISSN 1547-4127, ISBN-13: 978-0-323-70902-6

Editor: John Vassallo (j.vassallo@elsevier.com)
Developmental Editor: Laura Fisher

Thoracic Surgery Clinics (ISSN 1547-4127) is published quarterly by Elsevier Inc., 360 Park Avenue South, New York, NY 10010-1710. Months of publication are February, May, August, and November. Business and editorial offices: 1600 John F. Kennedy Boulevard, Suite 1800, Philadelphia, PA 19103-2899. Periodicals postage paid at New York, NY, and additional mailing offices. Subscription prices are $382.00 per year (US individuals), $585.00 per year (US institutions), $100.00 per year (US students), $460.00 per year (Canadian individuals), $757.00 per year (Canadian institutions), $225.00 per year (Canadian and international students), $475.00 per year (international individuals), and $757.00 per year (international institutions). Foreign air speed delivery is included in all Clinics' subscription prices. All prices are subject to change without notice. **POSTMASTER:** Send address changes to Thoracic Surgery Clinics, Elsevier Health Sciences Division, Subscription Customer Service, 3251 Riverport Lane, Maryland Heights, MO 63043. **Customer Service (orders, claims, online, change of address): Telephone: 1-800-654-2452 (U.S. and Canada); 314-447-8871 (outside U.S. and Canada). Fax: 314-447-8029. E-mail: journalscustomerservice-usa@elsevier.com (for print support); journalsonlinesupport-usa@elsevier.com (for online support).**

Reprints. For copies of 100 or more, of articles in this publication, please contact Commercial Rights Department, Elsevier Inc., 360 Park Avenue South, New York, NY 10010-1710. Tel: 212-633-3874; Fax: 212-633-3820; E-mail: reprints@elsevier.com.

Thoracic Surgery Clinics is covered in *MEDLINE/PubMed (Index Medicus), EMBASE/Excerpta Medica, Science Citation Index Expanded (SciSearch®), Journal Citation Reports/Science Edition,* and *Current Contents®/Clinical Medicine.*

Contributors

CONSULTING EDITOR

M. BLAIR MARSHALL, MD, FACS
Associate Chief for Quality and Safety, Division
of Thoracic Surgery; Brigham and Women's
Hospital; Associate Professor of Surgery,
Harvard Medical School, Boston,
Massachusetts

EDITORS

INDERPAL S. SARKARIA, MD, FACS
Vice Chairman, Clinical Affairs, Director,
Thoracic Robotic Surgery, Co-Director,
Esophageal and Lung Surgery Institute,
Department of Cardiothoracic Surgery,
University of Pittsburgh Medical Center,
University of Pittsburgh School of Medicine,
Pittsburgh, Pennsylvania

ABBAS EL-SAYED ABBAS, MD, MS, FACS
Professor and Vice Chair, Surgeon-in-Chief,
Department of Thoracic Medicine and Surgery,
Division of Thoracic Surgery, Section Chief,
Section of Thoracic Surgery, Lewis Katz
School of Medicine, Temple University,
Department of Surgical Oncology, Fox Chase
Cancer Center, Philadelphia, Pennsylvania

AUTHORS

ABBAS EL-SAYED ABBAS, MD, MS, FACS
Professor and Vice Chair, Surgeon-in-Chief,
Department of Thoracic Medicine and Surgery,
Division of Thoracic Surgery, Section Chief,
Section of Thoracic Surgery, Lewis Katz
School of Medicine, Temple University,
Department of Surgical Oncology, Fox Chase
Cancer Center, Philadelphia, Pennsylvania

GHULAM ABBAS, MD, MHCM, FACS
Chief, Division of Thoracic Surgery, WVU
Medicine, Morgantown, West Virginia

KAMIL A. ABBAS
West Virginia University Honors College,
Morgantown, West Virginia

OMAR AWAIS, DO
Chief of Thoracic Surgery, UPMC Mercy,
Department of Cardiothoracic Surgery,
University of Pittsburgh Medical Center,
Pittsburgh, Pennsylvania

NICHOLAS BAKER, MD
Department of Cardiothoracic Surgery,
University of Pittsburgh Medical Center,
Pittsburgh, Pennsylvania

CHARLES T. BAKHOS, MD, MS, FACS
Associate Professor, Department of Thoracic
Medicine and Surgery, Lewis Katz School of
Medicine, Temple University, Temple
University Hospital, Philadelphia,
Pennsylvania

NEIL W. BRISTER, PhD, MD
Professor, Department of Anesthesiology,
Temple University Hospital, Philadelphia,
Pennsylvania

ERNEST G. CHAN, MD, MPH
Integrated Cardiothoracic Surgical Resident,
Department of Cardiothoracic Surgery,
University of Pittsburgh Medical Center,
Pittsburgh, Pennsylvania

SARAH CHOI, MD
Resident, Department of Thoracic and
Cardiovascular Surgery, Cleveland Clinic
Foundation, Cleveland, Ohio

SUBRATO J. DEB, MD, FACS, FCCP
Professor, Section Chief, Thoracic and Foregut
Surgery, Division of Thoracic and
Cardiovascular Surgery, Department of
Surgery, University of Oklahoma Health
Sciences Center, Director of Thoracic
Oncology, The University of Oklahoma
Stephenson Cancer Center, Oklahoma City,
Oklahoma

ANKIT DHAMIJA, MD
CT Surgery Fellow, Department of
Cardiovascular and Thoracic Surgery, WVU
Medicine, Morgantown, West Virginia

CHIGOZIRIM N. EKEKE, MD
Department of Cardiothoracic Surgery,
University of Pittsburgh Medical Center,
Pittsburgh, Pennsylvania

BRADLEY HAMMOND, DO
Assistant Professor, Department of
Anesthesiology, Temple University Hospital,
Philadelphia, Pennsylvania

MATTHEW G. HARTWIG, MD, MHS
Associate Professor of Surgery, Program
Director, Minimally Invasive Thoracic Surgery
Fellowship, Division of Thoracic Surgery, Duke
University Health System, Durham, North
Carolina

JEREMIAH A. HAYANGA, MD
Associate Professor, Department of
Cardiovascular and Thoracic Surgery, WVU
Medicine, Morgantown, West Virginia

TARYNE A. IMAI, MD
Assistant Professor of Surgery, Division of
Thoracic Surgery, Cedars-Sinai Medical
Center, Los Angeles, California

TATIANA KAZAKOVA, MD
Resident, Department of Family Medicine,
Jefferson Health NE, Philadelphia,
Pennsylvania

ANNE-SOPHIE LALIBERTE, MD, FRCSC
Esophageal Fellow, Division of Thoracic
Surgery, Swedish Medical Center, Seattle,
Washington

RYAN LEVY, MD
Assistant Professor of Cardiothoracic Surgery,
Chief, Thoracic Surgery, Department of
Cardiothoracic Surgery, UPMC Passavant,
Pittsburgh, Pennsylvania

**BRIAN E. LOUIE, MD, MHA, MPH, FRCSC,
FACS**
Director, Thoracic Research and Education,
Executive Medical Director/Surgical Chair,
Swedish Digestive Health Institute, Division of
Thoracic Surgery, Swedish Medical Center,
Seattle, Washington

JAMES D. LUKETICH, MD
Chairman, Department of Cardiothoracic
Surgery, University of Pittsburgh Medical
Center, Pittsburgh, Pennsylvania

SUDISH MURTHY, MD, PhD
Section Head, Department of Thoracic and
Cardiovascular Surgery, Cleveland Clinic
Foundation, Cleveland, Ohio

SARA NAJMEH, MD
Thoracic Surgery Fellow, Duke University,
Durham, North Carolina

SHREY P. PATEL, MD
Cardiothoracic Surgery Resident, Department
of Surgery, Lewis Katz School of Medicine,
Temple University, Temple University Hospital,
Philadelphia, Pennsylvania

ARJUN PENNATHUR, MD
Associate Professor, Department of
Cardiothoracic Surgery, University of
Pittsburgh Medical Center, Pittsburgh,
Pennsylvania

ROMAN V. PETROV, MD, PhD, FACS
Assistant Professor, Department of Thoracic
Medicine and Surgery, Division of Thoracic
Surgery, Lewis Katz School of Medicine,
Temple University, Department of Surgical
Oncology, Fox Chase Cancer Center,
Philadelphia, Pennsylvania

SIVA RAJA, MD, PhD
Staff, Department of Thoracic and
Cardiovascular Surgery, Cleveland
Clinic Foundation, Cleveland,
Ohio

JAMES MATTHEW REINERSMAN, MD, FACS
Assistant Professor, Division of Thoracic and Cardiovascular Surgery, Department of Surgery, University of Oklahoma Health Sciences Center, Oklahoma City, Oklahoma

INDERPAL S. SARKARIA, MD, FACS
Vice Chairman, Clinical Affairs, Director, Thoracic Robotic Surgery, Co-Director, Esophageal and Lung Surgery Institute, Department of Cardiothoracic Surgery, University of Pittsburgh Medical Center, University of Pittsburgh School of Medicine, Pittsburgh, Pennsylvania

ASHISH C. SINHA, MD, PhD, MBA
Professor, Department of Anesthesiology, Temple University Hospital, Philadelphia, Pennsylvania

HARMIK J. SOUKIASIAN, MD
Professor of Surgery, Chief, Division of Thoracic Surgery, Cedars-Sinai Medical Center, Los Angeles, California

STACEY SU, MD
Assistant Professor, Department of Surgical Oncology, Fox Chase Cancer Center, Philadelphia, Pennsylvania

CHAD TALAREK, MD
Assistant Professor, Department of Anesthesiology, Temple University Hospital, Philadelphia, Pennsylvania

ANDREW TANG, MD
Resident, Department of Thoracic and Cardiovascular Surgery, Cleveland Clinic Foundation, Cleveland, Ohio

MATTHEW VERCAUTEREN, PA-C
Department of Cardiothoracic Surgery, University of Pittsburgh Medical Center, Pittsburgh, Pennsylvania

TADEUSZ D. WITEK, MD
Department of Cardiothoracic Surgery, University of Pittsburgh Medical Center, Pittsburgh, Pennsylvania

Contents

Paraesophageal hernia repair is a technically challenging operation. Factors that influence morbidity of the operation include the timing of the operation, surgical approach, and patient factors. Medical complications are the most common and usually are respiratory or cardiac related. Perforation, subcutaneous emphysema, pneumothorax, shortened esophagus, and presence of a large hernia all complicate paraesophageal hernia repair. Various strategies of intraoperative management are described. Management of leaks and perforations identified postoperatively are dictated by the clinical status of the patient. Early identification and expeditious intervention are paramount in the overall management of complications.

Paraesophageal hernia represents a complex surgical problem involving significant distortion of the anatomy and function of the esophagus, stomach, gastroesophageal junction, mediastinum, lungs, and heart. Surgeons operating in the area must have deep understanding of the normal anatomy and pathologic derangements in patients with paraesophageal hernias. This article describes the normal anatomy and anatomic abnormalities in application to the various approaches used in the surgical repair of a paraesophageal hernia.

 Video content accompanies this article at http://www.thoracic.theclinics.com.

The surgical approach to giant paraesophageal hernia repair has evolved considerably, from an open approach to minimally invasive approaches. Laparoscopic and robotic-assisted approaches to giant paraesophageal hernia have been considered safe and are associated with less morbidity and mortality. Limited data exist comparing the efficacy between laparoscopic and robotic-assisted giant paraesophageal hernia repairs, but the benefits of robotic surgery include superior optics and freedom of motion, thus allowing surgeons to accomplish the key points in a successful repair without compromising patient outcomes.

Gastroesophageal reflux disease (GERD) is common in the morbidly obese population, and hiatal hernias are encountered in 20% to 52% of patients. Primary surgical repair of hiatal hernias, in particular the paraesophageal type, is associated with a higher recurrence rate in obese patients. Concomitant weight loss surgery may be advisable. Combined sleeve gastrectomy and paraesophageal hiatal hernia repair is feasible but can induce or worsen preexisting GERD. A Roux-en-Y gastric bypass offers advantages of more pronounced excess weight loss and better symptom control, albeit with a potentially higher rate of morbidity compared with paraesophageal hernia repair alone or sleeve gastrectomy.

Failure to recognize a short esophagus during paraesophageal hernia repair can lead to poor functional outcomes and increased recurrence rates. Diagnosis is usually done intraoperatively when less than 2 to 3 cm of esophagus lie in the intraabdominal position. If aggressive esophageal mediastinal mobilization is unable to lengthen the esophagus, the surgeon should perform an esophageal lengthening procedure. A modified Collis gastroplasty is most commonly used and can be performed through a variety of transabdominal or transthoracic approaches. These procedures are safe, durable, and associated with good long-term outcomes. Patient selection and safe surgical technique are key in avoiding complications.

The introduction of minimally invasive techniques to the field of foregut surgery has revolutionized the surgical approach to giant paraesophageal hernia repair. Laparoscopy has become the standard approach in patients with giant paraesophageal hernia because it has been shown to be safe and is associated with lower morbidity and mortality when compared with various open approaches. Specifically, it has been associated with decreased intraoperative blood loss, decreased complications, and reduced hospital length of stay. This is despite a rise in comorbid conditions associated with this patient population. This article describes our operative approach to laparoscopic giant paraesophageal hernia repair.

The assessment of outcome after paraesophageal repair is difficult and complex. There is a wide range of reported outcomes that are not consistently defined. The focus of this article is on short-term ($\leq$5 years) and long-term (>5 year) outcomes after laparoscopic paraesophageal repair and reviews key patient-reported outcomes (gastroesophageal reflux disease [GERD]–related and non–GERD-related symptoms), radiologic recurrence, additional therapy, and objective measurements. Overall, patients reported an excellent improvement in their quality of life after repair that remains durable. Recurrences are lower when axial and radial tension is addressed. Reoperative surgery is infrequent.

Giant paraesophageal hernias can present as an asymptomatic incidentally detected paraesophageal hernia to an emergent gastric volvulus with concern for ischemia. In the acute setting, the preoperative evaluation aims to determine the extent of complications from gastric volvulus. In the elective setting, preoperative testing defines the gastroesophageal anatomy and function to select the optimal operation. Through thoughtful preoperative evaluation, the best operative approach can be tailored to each patient.

THORACIC SURGERY CLINICS

FORTHCOMING ISSUES

February 2020
Nonintubated Thoracic Surgery
Vincenzo Ambrogi and Tommaso Claudio
Mineo, *Editors*

May 2020
**Advances in Systemic Therapy for Non-Small
Cell Lung Cancer**
Jessica Donington and Jyoti Patel, *Editors*

August 2020
**Peri-operative Management of the Thoracic
Patient**
Virginia R. Litle and Robert J. Canelli, *Editors*

RECENT ISSUES

August 2019
**Thoracic Surgical Education: Current and
Future Strategies**
Edward D. Verrier, *Editor*

May 2019
Thymectomy for Myasthenia Gravis
Joshua R. Sonett, *Editor*

February 2019
**Surgery for Pulmonary Mycobacterial
Disease**
John D. Mitchell, *Editor*

SERIES OF RELATED INTEREST

Surgical Clinics
http://www.surgical.theclinics.com

Surgical Oncology Clinics
http://www.surgonc.theclinics.com

Advances in Surgery
http://www.advancessurgery.com

THE CLINICS ARE AVAILABLE ONLINE!
Access your subscription at:
www.theclinics.com

Preface

Paraesophageal Hernia Repair: A Still-Evolving Operation in Pursuit of Perfection

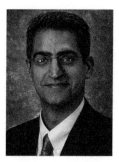
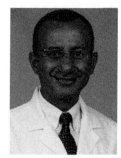

Inderpal S. Sarkaria, MD, FACS Abbas El-Sayed Abbas, MD, MS, FACS

Editors

We are pleased to present this issue of *Thoracic Surgery Clinics* dedicated to the surgical repair of paraesophageal hernias. Over the decades, our understanding and approach to the management of patients with substantial transhiatal herniation of the stomach and other abdominal viscera into the chest have changed significantly, while simultaneously still adhering to the traditional principles of repair that have stood the test of time. Traditionally approached from the chest by open thoracotomy, abdominal approaches have become the dominant route of repair, with minimally invasive laparoscopic approaches being the route of choice for many surgeons. Robotic approaches have increased in popularity as well, further increasing the operative choices afforded surgeons in caring for this disease.

While many (including the editors) would purport this operative evolution has decreased the morbidity of these operations over time, it would be difficult to argue against the position that proven routes of recurrence and failure still plague our patients to a significant degree. Rates of treatment failures in the form of recurrent herniation or symptomatic reflux continue to be significant sources of morbidity. Also, while often mistakenly thought of as a "simple" hernia repair, practitioners performing these operations come to appreciate the inherent complexity and potential difficulty of these operations in which anatomy can be significantly distorted, and adequate exposure and visualization can be difficult to create and maintain. Furthermore, in these "benign" cases, the simultaneous goal of preserving normal anatomic structures while restoring normal anatomic relationships can prove challenging, as opposed to the resective and exenterative nature of oncologic thoracic surgery. While largely adhering to a set of prime principles, these challenges have otherwise given rise to a rich range of operative approaches,

Thorac Surg Clin 29 (2019) xi–xii
https://doi.org/10.1016/j.thorsurg.2019.08.002
1547-4127/19/© 2019 Published by Elsevier Inc.

technique, and opinion regarding best practices in these cases.

In this issue, we are grateful to have had a truly expert faculty contribute their time and effort to presenting these topics and issues through the selected set of articles. While the articles have been developed to represent relatively unique topics pertinent to these operations, many of the primary principles and tenets of surgery and management are clearly reinforced throughout the readings. The reader will no doubt also find subtle (and sometimes less subtle!) differences in opinion by equally recognized experts in the field. I would urge the reader to approach these articles with the understanding that this speaks to the still-evolving nature of these operations, and the continuing pursuit of surgical perfection to a challenging and complex disease process.

It has been a privilege to work with the authors in assembling this focused issue on paraesophageal hernia repair, and we sincerely hope you enjoy the readings presented.

With warm regards,

Inderpal S. Sarkaria, MD, FACS
Department of Cardiothoracic Surgery
University of Pittsburgh Medical Center and
University of Pittsburgh School of Medicine
5200 Centre Avenue, Suite 715.27
Pittsburgh, PA 15232, USA

Abbas El-Sayed Abbas, MD, MS, FACS
Thoracic Medicine and Surgery
Section of Thoracic Surgery
Lewis Katz School of Medicine
Medicine Education & Research Building
3500 North Broad Street
Philadelphia, PA 19140, USA

E-mail addresses:
sarkariais@upmc.edu (I.S. Sarkaria)
abbas.abbas@tuhs.temple.edu (A.E.-S. Abbas)

Management of Complications in Paraesophageal Hernia Repair

Taryne A. Imai, MD, Harmik J. Soukiasian, MD*

KEYWORDS

- Paraesophageal hernia repair complications • Esophageal and gastric perforation
- Carbon dioxide insufflation complications • Collis gastroplasty • Hiatal hernia

KEY POINTS

- Paraesophageal hernia is a disease of the elderly, who are likely to have preexisting comorbidities; therefore, complications of repair tend to be medical.
- Drainage, restoration of mucosal integrity, antibiotics, and early initiation of nutritional support are tenets of management for perforation and leaks.
- Endoscopic treatments of perforations identified postoperatively have revolutionized management.
- With the adoption of laparoscopic paraesophageal hernia repairs, complications of carbon dioxide insufflation, such as subcutaneous emphysema and pneumothorax, are common.
- Management of the shortened esophagus and closure of the large hiatus associated with paraesophageal hernias remain controversial.

INTRODUCTION AND OVERALL PREVALENCE OF COMPLICATIONS

Paraesophageal hernias represent 5% to 10% of all hiatal hernias.[1] They are defined as greater than one-third of the stomach herniated into the mediastinum.[2] Postoperative complications develop in 3% to 45% of patients undergoing paraesophageal hernia repair.[1] Operative mortality rates have been reported to range from 0% to 3.7%.[2–5]

Most common complications after paraesophageal hernia repair tend to be medical. Respiratory-related complications include pneumonia, pulmonary embolism, and acute respiratory distress syndrome. Postoperative atrial fibrillation, myocardial infarction, and congestive heart failure are common cardiac complications. Additionally, ileus, acute renal failure, and urinary tract infections are prevalent complications.[2–4]

The incidence of complications that require reoperation within 30 days ranges from 1.6% to 4.9%.[1,2] A majority of these cases are due to postoperative leak, perioperative hernia recurrence, visceral injury, bleeding, obstructing fundoplication, or small bowel obstruction.

FACTORS CONTRIBUTING TO COMPLICATIONS
Timing of Surgery

Timing of surgical repair of paraesophageal hernias remains controversial. Repair on diagnosis irrespective of symptoms has been recommended to avoid potential life-threatening complications resulting from gastric torsion with subsequent ischemia, gangrene, perforation, and massive bleeding.[6] These complications have an overall mortality of 26% and an annual incidence ranging

Disclosure: The authors have nothing to disclose.
Division of Thoracic Surgery, Cedars-Sinai Medical Center, 8631 West 3rd Street, Suite 240E, Los Angeles, CA 90048, USA
* Corresponding author.
E-mail address: Harmik.Soukiasian@cshs.org

Thorac Surg Clin 29 (2019) 351–358
https://doi.org/10.1016/j.thorsurg.2019.07.009
1547-4127/19/© 2019 Elsevier Inc. All rights reserved.

from 0.7% to 7% of patients with paraesophageal hernias.[6–9] The pooled annual probability of requiring emergency surgery is estimated to be 1.16% per year, with a lifetime risk of 18% at age 65 years.[10] Some investigators have recommended elective repair only when patients are symptomatic, presenting with dysphagia, shortness of breath, persistent vomiting, chest discomfort or pain, and anemia.[10] Once symptoms develop, the annual probability of symptom progression is estimated to be 13.87% (8.15%–21.77%).[10] There is a significant difference in mortality rates for emergency versus elective paraesophageal hernia repair, with 17% for emergency surgery versus 1.38% for elective surgery.[10] Organ resection also may be necessary in 6.4% of patients undergoing emergency surgery.[10]

Surgical Approach

Operations for paraesophageal hernias are technically challenging and are associated with higher morbidity in comparison to other operations for benign esophageal disease. A standard approach to repair was transabdominal via an upper midline laparotomy. Currently, laparoscopic repairs have been accepted as a safe approach and are now more common. Outcomes of open and laparoscopic paraesophageal hernia repair have been compared. Although intraoperative complication rates are similar for both approaches (11% laparoscopic vs 12% open), the laparoscopic approach has a lower overall morbidity with fewer postoperative complications (28% laparoscopic vs 60% open).[4,11] Lower 30-day mortality also has been demonstrated in the laparoscopic group.[4] Many benefits of laparoscopic paraesophageal hernia repair have been described and include shorter operative time reported in later series, less blood loss, shorter length of hospital stay (3 days vs 9 days), decreased postoperative pain medication use, and shorter time to oral intake (1.13 days vs 6.1 days).[4,12,13] Conversion to open rates are low, ranging from 1.5% to 9.1%, and were due to bleeding, perforation, adhesions, or inability to reduce the hernia.[1] Furthermore, paraesophageal hernia repairs are notorious for high rates of recurrence. A comparison of recurrence rates by surgical approach reports higher recurrence with laparoscopy compared with open (42% vs 15%, respectively).[3]

Patient Factors

Patients diagnosed with paraesophageal hernia generally are older than patients with other benign esophageal diseases requiring surgery. Advanced age, with its inherent association of comorbidities,

contributes to increased mortality and morbidity of paraesophageal hernia repair. Of those patients undergoing surgery, most series report median age ranging from 63 years to 75 years old.[1,2] Advanced age has been demonstrated to influence postoperative morbidity and mortality, because patients older than 70 years are twice as likely to have complications compared with those younger than 70.[14] Preexisting comorbidities, defined by the American Society of Anesthesiologists (ASA) score, also influence morbidity. Although higher ASA scores increase postoperative complication rates, mortality is not affected.[14]

The type of hernia also can influence postoperative morbidity. Type 2 hernias have been reported to have a complication rate of 9.9%, type 3 hernias 11.1%, and, not surprisingly, type 4 hernias were associated with the highest complication rate of 23.3%.[14] This is not surprising that repair of type 4 hernias is the most challenging, because it is most difficult to reduce, includes presence of other visceral organs within the hernia sac, and has the largest hiatal defect to close. Additionally, patients older than 70 years presented with a higher incidence of type 4 hernias compared with patients younger than 70 years.[14]

Prediction of Complications

Because indications and timing of operative management for paraesophageal hernia remain controversial, prediction models for morbidity and mortality may help guide treatment decisions. The University of Pittsburgh established a clinical prediction model based on the outcomes of approximately 1000 patients undergoing paraesophageal hernia repair.[15] Older age at operation, lower body mass index, and larger hernia were associated with increased major postoperative morbidity. Perioperative mortality was increased and influenced by nonelective setting, age 80 or greater, lower body mass index, history of congestive heart failure, cerebral vascular incident, dementia, pulmonary disease, peptic ulcer disease, and malignancy within the past 5 years. Prediction models may be most applicable in treatment decisions for patients who are mildly symptomatic, by weighing the risks and benefits of proceeding with an operation.

IATROGENIC PERFORATION

Perforation is a known complication of paraesophageal hernia repair and can be due to many mechanisms. Injury can occur intraoperatively during extensive mediastinal periesophageal dissection and mobilization required to acquire adequate esophageal length. Difficulties in reducing the intrathoracic stomach can lead to traction injuries. Passage of the bougie during Nissen fundoplication or Collis gastroplasty also may cause perforation. Delayed perforation recognized postoperatively may be due to devascularization of the esophagus during extensive mediastinal dissection, which can lead to ischemia and subsequent perforation. Other mechanisms of delayed perforation may be a result of postoperative suture pull-through. Management of perforations includes a variety of procedures. Despite the type of procedure required, however, the following cardinal principles of perforation management should be upheld:

1. Prevent and control mediastinal and peritoneal contamination—adequate and appropriate drain placement
2. Control the leak by restoring mucosal integrity—primary repair, stenting, clipping, and so forth
3. Infection control—broad spectrum antibiotics and antifungals
4. Early initiation of nutritional support—parenteral nutrition and enteral nutrition

Intraoperative Management of Perforations

A large retrospective series from Washington University reviewed esophageal and gastric perforations during laparoscopic foregut surgery.[16] Perforations during laparoscopic paraesophageal hernia repair occurred in 1.8% of cases, which was higher than during antireflux surgery (1%) but lower than in Heller myotomy cases (3.3%). Of the 7 cases of iatrogenic perforations during paraesophageal hernia repair, 2 cases were esophageal and 5 were gastric. This distribution was consistent among the other foregut surgeries, where most perforations were located on the stomach. The mechanism of perforation for laparoscopic paraesophageal hernia repair were predominantly due to traction (43%), followed by suture placement, bougie insertion, and thermal injury. To prevent perforations due to traction, mobilization of the hernia sac prior to reducing the stomach has been suggested. In addition, a majority of perforations during paraesophageal hernia repair were recognized intraoperatively (71.4%) versus postoperatively (28.6%).

When iatrogenic perforations are recognized and treated intraoperatively, they often do not negatively affect the outcomes. Perforations identified postoperatively, however, are associated with increased postoperative complications, longer hospital stays, and more interventions. Therefore, the most important principle in managing iatrogenic perforations is early recognition and treatment intraoperatively, if possible. Investigational methods to identify potential intraoperative perforations include using a nasogastric tube to fill the distal esophageal lumen with methylene blue or utilizing upper endoscopy to identify possible perforations by air insufflation with the esophagus or stomach under water. When iatrogenic perforations are recognized, they can be closed with 1 or 2 layers, or, if on the stomach, a linear stapler can also be used. Once closed, a wrap of the stomach can be used to buttress or reinforce esophageal perforation repairs. Either a Dor fundoplication or partial posterior fundoplication can be performed depending on the location of the perforation. At the completion of the operation, a drain should be placed at the site of repair and postoperatively a contrast swallow study may be performed prior to feeding. At the authors' institution, other methods used to investigate the integrity of the repair include checking drain amylase levels and drinking colored liquids.

Management of Delayed Perforations

Iatrogenic perforations may be identified postoperatively, by the presence of tachycardia, fever, and leukocytosis, or radiographically with contrast swallow studies. In patients with delayed identification of iatrogenic perforation, management is dictated by the clinical picture of the patient. Patients presenting with peritonitis or transabdominal sepsis and who are acutely ill may require urgent reoperation to attempt primary closure of the perforation with buttressed repair and drainage. Often, due to the friability of the tissue, primary repair cannot be performed. Drains may be placed adjacent to the perforation to widely drain the leak and provide source control. Diversion may be required for complicated cases involving elderly, malnourished, septic patients on vasopressors or those who are undiagnosed for several days. Additionally, diversion may be required when the surrounding tissue is severely edematous, inflamed, or ischemic.

Removable covered stents have become popular and revolutionized management of esophageal perforations. Utilizing stents as a treatment option often avoids highly morbid reoperations and need for esophageal diversion. Stents are deployed endoscopically and allow for early oral nutrition once the leak is sealed.[17] Initially, earlier generation stents were not ideal for benign esophageal pathology because they were not removable. Now with the advent of covered stents, which prevent tissue in-growth, stents are easily removable and an acceptable treatment option in benign esophageal disease. Although stents provide numerous advantages, they also can be problematic. Common issues with stents include stent migration, reflux, patient discomfort or pain, difficult removal, and injury or erosion to adjacent structures. Stent migration has been reported in 16% to 37.5% of cases, with most patients requiring endoscopic intervention.[17–20] Migration is more common particularly with perforations because the esophagus does not have a stricture or obstruction to hold the stent in place, as is the case with malignant disease. To prevent stent migration, longer and wider bore stents may be selected or anchoring the stent with endoclips has been described.[20] Although stents offer treatment advantages for postoperative perforations, adjunctive operations, such as decortications, wash outs, muscle or tissue flap reinforcement, or drain placement, may still be necessary. Once a stent is confirmed to be appropriately placed, a contrast study should be done to confirm appropriate seal and no leakage prior to initiating oral intake. To facilitate removal, esophageal stents should be extracted, and healing evaluated within 30 days. A contrast study should be performed after stent removal. If the leak persists, another stent may be deployed and assessed after another 30-day period.[17]

In addition to stents, several endoluminal interventions may provide advantageous options for the treatment of foregut perforations identified postoperatively.[20,21] Endoscopic closure of perforations with clips or sutures can successfully close esophageal and gastric perforations less than 2 cm.[20] Clips are classified as either through the scope clips or over the scope clips, both requiring the tissue surrounding the edges of the perforation to be compliant and viable. Indurated or friable tissue may limit the success of clips. A systematic review of endoclip closure for esophageal perforations demonstrated successful closure in perforations ranging from 3 mm to 25 mm in length.[22] The median time to closure of a perforation after clip application was 18 days. The only factor that predicted closure was the duration of perforation and, for every 10-day increase in the duration of a perforation, healing time increased by 7 days. Age of the patient and size of perforation were not found to be predictors of closure time. Limitations to endoscopic clips are due to wingspan and restricted ability to grab tissue and, therefore, they should not be used for larger perforations. Stents or endoscopic suturing should be considered for perforations greater than 2 cm. Endoscopic suturing requires a single-use disposable device mounted on the end of a gastroscope and can be applied in a continuous or interrupted fashion.

Perforations ranging in length from 25mm to 50mm can be successfully endoscopically closed.[23]

Endoluminal vacuum (EVAC) therapy also has been used recently to heal leaks and perforations successfully. The vacuum mechanism has added benefits of providing source control by the ability to use continuous suction to clear bacterial contamination as well as to perform serial débridement of the leak cavity. Healing is promoted by secondary intention. The endoscope first visualizes the leak or perforation site; the cavity is irrigated, débrided, and then sized. A 16-French nasogastric tube is placed through the nares and retrieved through the mouth. An endosponge is sutured to the tip of the nasogastric tube. The endoscope with the rat tooth grasper in the working channel then guides the endosponge down the esophagus and seats the sponge into the site of perforation. The nasogastric tube is then connected to the vacuum system to a pressure of 70 mm Hg to 125 mm Hg. Sponges are changed every 3 days to 5 days. Baylor University Medical Center reported 86% success of healing perforations with EVAC therapy.[24] Complete closure of esophageal perforations occurred in a mean of 27.1 days, whereas gastric perforations healed after a mean of 29.7 days. EVAC therapy had a 0% 30-day mortality and there were no complications directly related to endosponge use. A disadvantage to EVAC therapy is the need for multiple endoscopies to exchange endosponges. In the first meta-analysis comparing EVAC therapy with stenting for the treatment of esophageal leaks and perforations, vacuum therapy demonstrated a higher success rate of healing, shorter treatment duration, decreased incidence of major complications, and decreased in-hospital mortality.[25]

COMPLICATIONS OF CARBON DIOXIDE INSUFFLATION

With the acceptance and popularity of laparoscopic paraesophageal hernia repairs, complications of CO_2 insufflation are more prevalent. Subcutaneous emphysema and pneumothorax are common occurrences intraoperatively and, in most cases, can be managed without intervention.

Subcutaneous Emphysema

Risk factors for the development of subcutaneous emphysema are end-tidal CO_2 greater than 50 mm Hg, the use of 6 or more laparoscopic ports, and operative time more than 200 minutes.[26] Additionally, insufflation of the preperitoneal space, trocar pull-out or malpositioning, and use of increased insufflation pressures also may result in subcutaneous emphysema. For the most part, subcutaneous emphysema usually can be tolerated without the need for intervention or interruption of surgery. If intervention is required, CO_2 insufflation can be released temporarily and minute ventilation increased to eliminate CO_2. The surgery then can be resumed with lower insufflation pressures.

Pneumothorax

Although subcutaneous emphysema alone may have no clinical sequelae, its presence can be indicative of pneumothorax. Spontaneous pneumothorax is a result of the equalization of pressures across the diaphragm and the high diffusion capacity of CO_2.[27] More commonly, the mechanism of pneumothorax often is a result of violating the mediastinal pleura or the diaphragm. The concern of a shortened esophagus associated with paraesophageal hernias has led to more aggressive and extensive mediastinal dissection, which also increases the propensity of pleural tears. Intraoperatively, the development of a pneumothorax may be indicated by increased airway pressures, increased end-tidal CO_2, decreased peripheral oxygen saturation, acute onset of hypotension, and tachycardia, or bradycardia.[26,28] Pneumothorax also is suspected with the presence of a floppy or bulging diaphragm, caused by the loss of negative intrathoracic pressure. The convex movement of the diaphragm with ventilations may obscure the view and exposure of the hiatus. To stabilize hemodynamics and restore the optimal view of the hiatus, intervention for the pneumothorax may be necessary. The pleural rent can be closed using a PDS Endoloop (Ethicon, Cincinnati, Ohio) or laparoscopic clips or repaired using a barbed suture if the defect is large. Additionally, inserting an intercostal drain can be performed to prevent clinical deterioration but may not be ideal, because it causes loss of pneumoperitoneum. With a drain in place, the operation sometimes can be continued by decreasing the insufflation pressure and increasing the insufflation rate of CO_2.[26] The use of positive end-expiratory pressure (PEEP) as an alternative to chest tube insertion has also been described. PEEP decreases the pressure gradient between the abdominal and pleural cavities during both inspiration and expiration, thus inflating the lung. The re-expansion of the lung with PEEP can mechanically seal or plug the pleural tear.[29] Given the multiple strategies employed to manage intraoperative pneumothorax, the need to convert to open surgery has become rare.

Postoperatively, a pneumothorax may be present on chest radiograph and often can be observed without placement of a chest tube, in a clinically stable asymptomatic patient. The pneumothorax actually is a capnothorax, acquired intraoperatively with CO_2 entering the pleural space. CO_2 is a highly absorbable and soluble gas. Therefore, the pneumothorax often spontaneously resolves on subsequent imaging without need for intervention.[30]

COMPLICATIONS DUE TO THE SHORTENED ESOPHAGUS

A majority of paraesophageal hernias are type 3, identified by the migration of the gastroesophageal junction above the diaphragm. A well-known complicating factor of type III paraesophageal hernias is the presence of a shortened esophagus and its association with high recurrence rates during surgical repair. Therefore, restoring the normal anatomic position of the gastroesophageal junction and obtaining adequate intra-abdominal esophageal length (2–2.5 cm below the hiatus) is an important component of paraesophageal hernia surgery. If an intra-abdominal position of the gastroesophageal junction cannot be restored, then an esophageal lengthening procedure, such as a Collis gastroplasty, may be required to release the axial tension caused by the shortened esophagus.[31–36]

When compared with patients undergoing straightforward fundoplication, patients requiring Collis gastroplasty have equivalent postoperative mortality, length of stay, and quality of life and no difference in recurrence.[35] As demonstrated by Nason and colleagues,[35] however, the Collis gastroplasty group did have a higher incidence of postoperative leaks compared with the fundoplication-only group (2.7% vs 0.6%, respectively). Additionally, the overall experience of the institution demonstrated that 88% of their postoperative leaks occurred in those patients who required a Collis gastroplasty. Therefore, for patients who require a Collis gastroplasty, a contrast swallow study is recommended prior to oral intake. If a leak is present, but contained, and the patient is not acutely ill, conservative management is appropriate. Patients should be drained appropriately, either leaving in the intraoperative drain or having a percutaneous drain placed. Additionally, antibiotics should be started, ceasing oral intake, and parenteral nutrition or enteral nutrition via a feeding tube initiated.[37] If the leak is not contained or the patient is clinically toxic, then surgical intervention may be necessary. Primary repair with buttressing by surrounding tissues, such as omentum, and wide drainage, should be performed. A decompressive gastrostomy tube and distal feeding access with a jejunostomy tube also should be considered.[37]

Minor complications after Collis gastroplasty also have been described. In an early analysis of a small series of patients who had undergone fundoplication with Collis gastroplasty, postoperative manometry, endoscopy, 24-hour pH test, and endoscopic Congo red staining were performed to examine acid secretion in the Collis segment. Although only 14% of patients had complaints of postoperative heartburn, 50% of patients were found to have significant acid secretion from functional parietal cells in the Collis segment and 36% had persistent esophagitis.[38] Therefore, the authors recommend that patients treated with Collis gastroplasty have close objective follow-up and maintenance acid-suppression therapy.

MANAGEMENT OF COMPLICATIONS DUE TO THE LARGE HIATUS

The high rate of recurrence with paraesophageal hernia repairs has been reported to be in excess of 50% on median follow-up, ranging from 17 months to 58 months.[3,39] Recurrence is a common complication of the operation, due to the difficulty and inability of performing a durable tension-free repair of a large hiatus. The best technique to repair the hiatal hernia remains a controversial component of the operation. Primary suture crural reapproximation with preservation of the peritoneal lining over the crura is preferred and performed in a majority of cases.[2] Additionally, extensive mobilization of the crura from the surrounding gastrophrenic and splenophrenic attachments also has been advocated.[40] If the peritoneal lining is compromised or if the hiatal defect is large, reinforced repair with prosthetic mesh has been proposed. A meta-analysis comparing mesh versus suture repair demonstrates a reduced rate of recurrence with the use of mesh in short-term follow-up.[41] Currently, there is no consensus on the best method of performing a mesh repair. A variety of techniques, mesh shapes, and mesh types have been described in mesh repairs.[42,43] Although a mesh repair has been proposed as a solution to decrease the high recurrence rate of paraesophageal hernias, its use has not been routinely adopted due to the risk of serious complications related to the prosthesis.[41] Reported complication rates of mesh repairs range from 4.9% to 20%.[41,44] A multi-institutional case series described mesh complications after prosthetic reinforcement of hiatal closure.[45] Primary symptoms associated with mesh complications included dysphagia in the majority of patients, followed by chest pain, heartburn, weight loss, epigastric pain, and fever. Postoperative follow-up revealed complications of intraluminal esophageal mesh erosion, esophageal stenosis, mesh migration, hiatal stenosis, and dense local fibrosis.[41,45] To manage these complications, a majority of the patients required reoperation for mesh removal. A small subset of these patients required esophagectomy.[45]

Because the management of the large hiatal hernia continues to be controversial, Kang and colleagues[46] describes their experience using a pledgeted repair to prevent suture pull-through and reinforce crural reapproximation. Furthermore, if the peritoneal lining of the crura is damaged during dissection, a pledgeted repair may be necessary. The posterior hiatus is primarily reapproximated using sutures with Teflon pledgets on both sides of the crura. A majority of patients in this series were asymptomatic on postoperative follow-up (63%) and most were satisfied or very satisfied (83%). Additionally, the recurrence rate was 7% with a mean follow-up of 161 days.

Deliberate left pneumothorax induced by a small thoracostomy tube and carbon dioxide insufflation also has been described to facilitate closure of a large hiatus, thus avoiding the need for a mesh repair.[40] The pneumothorax causes the left hemidiaphragm to be floppy, which allows for tension-free suturing of the crura. Another maneuver to reduce crural tension utilizes relaxing incisions on the right hemidiaphragm, left hemidiaphragm, or both hemidiaphragms. To prevent phrenic nerve injury, incisions were not placed radially, but rather followed the inferior margin of the rib and out laterally.[47] To prevent herniation of abdominal contents into the chest, relaxing incisions should be covered with synthetic mesh. Biologic mesh has been used for right-sided relaxing incisions because the left lateral lobe of the liver may prevent diaphragmatic hernias.[48]

SUMMARY

Paraesophageal hernia repair is a technically challenging operation. Morbidity of the operation is influenced by the timing of the operation, surgical approach, and patient factors. Patients with paraesophageal hernia are generally older and have preexisting multiple comorbidities. Therefore, the most common complications tend to be medical and usually are respiratory related or cardiac related. Perforation, subcutaneous emphysema, pneumothorax, shortened esophagus, and presence of a large hernia all complicate paraesophageal hernia repair. Various strategies of intraoperative management have been described. For patients with leaks and perforations identified postoperatively, overall management includes drainage, source control, antibiotics, and initiation of nutrition. The decision to reoperate in these cases is dictated by the clinical status of the patient. Additionally, endoscopic interventions offer less invasive and effective treatment options for leaks and perforations. Early identification and expeditious intervention are paramount in the overall management of complications.

REFERENCES

1. Mehta S, Boddy A, Rhodes M. Review of outcome after laparoscopic paraesophageal hiatal hernia repair. Surg Laparosc Endosc Percutan Tech 2006; 16:301–6.
2. Luketich J, Nason K, Christie N, et al. Outcomes after a decade of laparoscopic giant paraesophageal hernia repair. J Thorac Cardiovasc Surg 2010; 139(2):395–404, 404.e1.
3. Hashemi M, Peters J, DeMeester T, et al. Laparoscopic repair of large type III hiatal hernia: objective follow-up reveals high recurrence rate. J Am Coll Surg 2000;190:553–60.
4. Schauer P, Ikramuddin S, McLaughlin R, et al. Comparison of laparoscopic versus open repair of paraesophageal hernia. Am J Surg 1998;176:659–65.
5. Altorki N, Yankelevitz D, Skinner D. Massive hiatal hernias: the anatomic basis of repair. J Thorac Cardiovasc Surg 1998;115:828–35.
6. Sihvo E, Salo J, Rasanen J, et al. Fatal complications of adult paraesophageal hernia: a population-based study. J Thorac Cardiovasc Surg 2009;137(2):419–24.
7. Skinner D, Belsey R. Surgical management of esophageal reflux and hiatus hernia: long-term results with 1,030 patients. J Thorac Cardiocasc Surg 1967;53:33–54.
8. Allen M, Trastek V, Deschamps C, et al. Intrathoracic stomach. Presentation and results of operation. J Thorac Cardiovasc Surg 1993;105:253–9.
9. Hallissey M, Ratliff D, Temple J, et al. Paraesophageal hiatus hernia: surgery for all ages. Ann R Coll Surg Engl 1992;74:23–5.
10. Stylopoulos N, Gazelle S, Rattner D. Paraesophageal hernias: operation or observation? Ann Surg 2002;236:492–501.
11. Mungo B, Molena D, Stem M, et al. Thirty-day outcomes of paraesophageal hernia repair using the NSQIP database: should laparoscopy be the standard of care? J Am Coll Surg 2014;219:229–36.
12. Zehetner J, DeMeester S, Ayazi S, et al. Laparoscopic versus open repair of paraesophageal hernia: the second decade. J Am Coll Surg 2011;212: 813–20.
13. Karmali S, McFadden S, Mitchell P, et al. Primary laparoscopic and open repair of paraesophageal hernias: a comparison of short-term outcomes. Dis Esophagus 2008;21:63–8.
14. Larusson H, Zingg U, Hahnloser D, et al. Predictive factors for morbidity and mortality in patients undergoing laparoscopic paraesophageal hernia repair: age, ASA score, and operation type influence morbidity. World J Surg 2009;33:980–5.
15. Ballian N, Luketich J, Levy R, et al. A clinical prediction rule for perioperative mortality and major morbidity after laparoscopic giant paraesophageal hernia repair. J Thorac Cardiovasc Surg 2013;145: 721–9.
16. Zhang L, Chang R, Matthews B, et al. Incidence, mechanisms, and outcomes of esophageal and gastric perforation during laparoscopic foregut surgery: a retrospective review of 1,223 foregut cases. Surg Endosc 2014;28:85–90.
17. Blackmon S, Santora R, Schwarz P, et al. Utility of removable esophageal covered self-expanding metal stents for leak and fistula management. Ann Thorac Surg 2010;89:931–7.
18. Ott C, Raitu N, Endlicher E, et al. Self-expanding Polyflex plastic stents in esophageal disease: various indications, complications, and outcomes. Surg Endosc 2007;21:889–96.
19. Sabharwal T, Hamady M, Chui S, et al. A randomized prospective comparison of the Flamingo Wallstent and Ultraflex stent for palliation of dysphagia associated with lower third esophageal carcinoma. Gut 2003;52:922–6.
20. Raju G. Endoscopic management of gastrointestinal leaks. Gastrointest Endosc Clin N Am 2007;17: 487–503.
21. Gomez-Esquivel R, Raju G. Endoscopic closure of acute esophageal perforations. Curr Gastroenterol Rep 2013;15:321.
22. Qadeer M, Dumot J, Vargo J, et al. Endoscopic clips for closing esophageal perforations: case report and pooled analysis. Gastrointest Endosc 2007;66: 605–11.
23. Sharaiha R, Kumta N, DeFilippis E, et al. A large multicenter experience with endoscopic suturing for management of gastrointestinal defects and stent anchorage in 122 patients: a retrospective review. J Clin Gastroenterol 2016;50:388–92.
24. Mencio M, Ontiveros E, Burdick J, et al. Use of novel technique to manage gastrointestinal leaks with endoluminal negative pressure: a single institution experience. Surg Endosc 2018;32:3349–56.
25. Rausa E, Asti A, Aiol A, et al. Comparison of endoscopic vacuum therapy versus endoscopic stenting for esophageal leaks: systematic review and meta-analysis. Dis Esophagus 2018;31:1–8.
26. Kaur R, Kohli S, Jain A, et al. Pneumothorax during laparoscopic repair of giant paraesophageal hernia. J Anaesthesiol Clin Pharmacol 2011;27:373–6.
27. Marcus D, Lau W, Swanstrom L. Carbon dioxide pneumothorax in laparoscopic surgery. Am J Surg 1996;171:464–6.

28. Falk G, D'Netto T, Phillips S, et al. Pneumothorax: laparoscopic intraoperative management during fundoplication facilitates management of cardiopulmonary instability and surgical exposure. J Laparoendosc Adv Surg Tech A 2018;28:1371–3.

29. Joris J, Chiche J, Lamy M. Pneumothorax during laparoscopic fundoplication: diagnosis and treatment with positive end-expiratory pressure. Anesth Analg 1995;81:993–1000.

30. Msezane L, Zorn K, Gofrit O, et al. Case report: conservative management of a large capnothorax following laparoscopic renal surgery. J Endourol 2008;21:1445–8.

31. Demeester S, Demeester T. Editorial comment: the short esophagus: going, going, gone? Surgery 2003;133(4):358–63.

32. Kalloor G, Deshpande A, Collis J. Observations on esophageal length. Thorax 1976;31(3):284–8.

33. Gozzetti G, Pilotti V, Spangaro M, et al. Pathophysiology and natural history of acquired short esophagus. Surgery 1987;102(3):507–14.

34. Puri V, Jacobsen K, Bell J, et al. Hiatal hernia repair with or without esophageal lengthening: is there a difference? Innovations 2013;8:341–7.

35. Nason K, Luketich J, Awais O, et al. Quality of life after Collis gastroplasty for short esophagus in patients with paraesophageal hernia. Ann Thorac Surg 2011;92:1854–61.

36. Swanstrom L, Marcus D, Galloway G. Laparoscopic Collis gastroplasty is the treatment of choice for the shortened esophagus. Am J Surg 1996;171:477–81.

37. Urschel J. Gastroesophageal leaks after antireflux operations. Ann Thorac Surg 1994;57:1229–32.

38. Jobe B, Horvath K, Swanstrom L. Postoperative function following laparoscopic Collis gastroplasty for shortened esophagus. Arch Surg 1998;133: 867–74.

39. Oelschlager B, Pellegrini C, Hunter J, et al. Biologic prosthesis to prevent recurrence after laparoscopic paraesophageal hernia repair: long-term follow-up from a multicenter, prospective, randomized trial. J Am Coll Surg 2011;213:461–8.

40. Tam V, Luketich J, Levy R, et al. Mesh cruroplasty in laparoscopic repair of paraesophageal hernias is not associated with better long-term outcomes compared to primary repair. Am J Surg 2017;214: 651–6.

41. Zhang C, Liu D, Li F, et al. Systematic review and meta-analysis of laparoscopic mesh versus suture repair of hiatus hernia: objective and subjective outcomes. Surg Endosc 2017;31:4913–22.

42. Frantzides C, Carlson M, Loizides S, et al. Hiatal hernia repair with mesh: a survey of SAGES members. Surg Endosc 2010;24(5):1017–24.

43. Pfluke J, Parker M, Bowers S, et al. Use of mesh for hiatal hernia repair: a survey of SAGES members. Surg Endosc 2012;26(7):1843–8.

44. Griffith P, Valenti V, Qurashi K, et al. Rejection of Gore-Tex mesh used in prosthetic cruroplasty. Int J Surg 2008;6:106–9.

45. Stadlhuber R, Sherif A, Mittal S, et al. Mesh complications after prosthetic reinforcement of hiatal closure: a 28-case series. Surg Endosc 2009;23: 1219–26.

46. Kang T, Urrego H, Gridley A, et al. Pledgeted repair of giant hiatal hernia provides excellent long-term results. J Laparoendosc Adv Surg Tech A 2014;24: 684–7.

47. Alicuben E, Worrell S, DeMeester S. Impact of crural relaxing incisions, Collis gastroplasty, and non-cross-linked human dermal mesh crural reinforcement on early hiatal hernia recurrence rates. J Am Coll Surg 2014;219:988–92.

48. Crespin O, Yates R, Martin A, et al. The use of crural relaxing incisions with biologic mesh reinforcement during laparoscopic repair of complex hiatal hernia. Surg Endosc 2016;30:2179–85.

Surgical Anatomy of Paraesophageal Hernias

Roman V. Petrov, MD, PhD[a,b,*], Stacey Su, MD[b], Charles T. Bakhos, MD, MS[a], Abbas El-Sayed Abbas, MD, MS[a,b]

KEYWORDS

- Hiatal hernia • Paraesophageal hernia • Surgical anatomy • Esophageal hiatus
- Gastroesophageal junction

KEY POINTS

- Incidence of paraesophageal hernias is increasing owing to the increased proportion of advanced age patients and clinicians' awareness.
- Minimally invasive, including robotic, surgical techniques are increasing in popularity and produce excellent results.
- Thorough understanding of anatomic relationship in paraesophageal hernias is required for successful surgical repair regardless of the surgical approach.

NORMAL ESOPHAGEAL ANATOMY

The esophagus is a tubular organ, approximately 25 cm long, which connects the hypopharynx to the stomach. Along its course, it traverses 3 body areas: the neck, the chest, and the abdomen (**Fig. 1**A). Accordingly, it is subdivided into 3 anatomic segments: cervical, thoracic, and abdominal.

The cervical segment of the esophagus starts at the hypopharynx, from which it is separated by the upper esophageal sphincter, at the level of the sixth cervical vertebra. The cervical esophagus extends down to the level of suprasternal notch. It is located directly behind and partially to the left of the trachea, in front of C6 and C7 vertebral bodies. Laterally, the esophagus is surrounded by the lower poles of the thyroid gland and the carotid sheaths. On the left side, the termination of the thoracic duct can be found entering the venous angle at the junction of the left internal jugular and subclavian veins.

The thoracic esophagus extends from the suprasternal notch to the diaphragmatic hiatus. It enters the chest through the thoracic inlet and is located initially in the superior and then the posterior mediastinum. The midesophagus deviates slightly to the right, usually passing behind the left mainstem bronchus and pericardium anterior to the prevertebral fascia of T1 though T10 vertebral bodies. Both vagus nerves accompany the esophagus throughout its course on each side. The descending thoracic aorta is located posteriorly and to the left, whereas the mediastinal pleura drapes over both sides of the esophagus.

The abdominal esophagus is a short segment of the organ, extending from the diaphragmatic hiatus at the level of T10 to the gastric cardia at the level of T11. After passing through the hiatus, the abdominal esophagus deviates to the left and enters the stomach, forming the gastroesophageal junction (GEJ). The descending aorta is located posterior to the GEJ, and the inferior vena cava is posterior and to the right. It is covered anteriorly by the left lobe of the liver.

In cross-section, the esophagus has 3 layers (mucosa, submucosa, and muscularis propria)

Dr. Abbas received honoraria from Boston Scientific and Intuitive. No disclosures for other authors.
[a] Department of Thoracic Medicine and Surgery, Division of Thoracic Surgery, Lewis Katz School of Medicine at Temple University, 3401 North Broad Street C-501, Philadelphia, PA 19140, USA; [b] Department of Surgical Oncology, Fox Chase Cancer Center, 333 Cottman Avenue C-312, Philadelphia, PA 19111, USA
* Corresponding author. Department of Thoracic Medicine and Surgery, Division of Thoracic Surgery, Lewis Katz School of Medicine at Temple University, 3401 North Broad Street C-501, Philadelphia, PA 19140.
E-mail address: Roman.Petrov@tuhs.temple.edu

Thorac Surg Clin 29 (2019) 359–368
https://doi.org/10.1016/j.thorsurg.2019.07.008
1547-4127/19/© 2019 Elsevier Inc. All rights reserved.

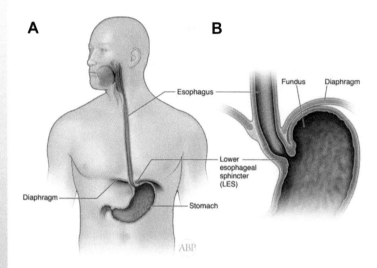

Fig. 1. Anatomy of the esophagus and GEJ. (*A*) Position of the esophagus, with its locations in the neck, chest, and abdomen. (*B*) Diaphragm, esophageal hiatus and gastroesophageal junction.

surrounded by the adventitia. After crossing through the hiatus, the esophagus is enveloped by the visceral peritoneum, forming a serosa. The muscularis propria, formed in the proximal third of the esophagus by striated muscle, is replaced by smooth muscle in the distal esophagus. It consists of an inner circular layer and outer longitudinal layer. The circular muscle fibers are arranged in a helical fashion, sometimes giving rise to a corkscrew appearance in many motility disorders.[1]

The blood supply to the esophagus is segmental. The cervical esophagus is supplied by branches of the inferior thyroid arteries, whereas the thoracic esophagus is supplied by small aortoesophageal arteries, in addition to branches from the bronchial and superior phrenic arteries. The abdominal esophagus receives blood supply from branches of the left gastric artery, the splenic artery, and the left inferior phrenic artery. Venous drainage forms a submucosal plexus, draining the cervical segment through the inferior thyroid veins and the thoracic esophagus through the azygos system into the superior vena cava. The lower thoracic and abdominal esophagus is drained into the portal system via the gastric veins. In cases of portal hypertension, these lower esophageal veins can dilate, forming esophageal varices.

The lymphatic drainage also starts at the submucosal plexus, forming lymphatic channels that drain into the regional lymph nodes. The deep cervical nodes receive lymph flow from the cervical and the upper thoracic esophagus. The paraesophageal lymph nodes of the superior and posterior mediastinum drain the thoracic segment. The lower thoracic segment and the abdominal esophagus drain into the celiac and perigastric lymph nodes. There is significant overlap in the lymphatic drainage between these segments.

The intrinsic nervous system is formed by the submucosal and the intramuscular neural plexi. Innervation to the esophagus is supplied by both vagus nerves, providing the parasympathetic control of esophageal wall motility, the esophageal sphincters, and glandular secretions. Sympathetic innervation is provided by the sympathetic chains and is mostly responsible for vasomotor effects and pain sensation. The vagus nerves arise in the medulla oblongata as the tenth cranial nerves and after exiting the skull base run on each side of the esophagus. They enter the chest via the thoracic inlet and travel caudally along the esophagus to the hiatus. Because of the embryologic clock-wise rotation of the lower foregut in the abdomen, the left vagus nerve becomes anterior, whereas the right vagus nerve lies posteriorly.[1,2]

STOMACH

The stomach is a J-shaped saccular expansion of the foregut, serving as a reservoir for the ingested food at the beginning of the digestive process (**Fig. 2**A). It receives the food bolus from the esophagus, via the GEJ, below the esophageal hiatus. It transitions into the duodenum at the pylorus. On the right, the concave edge of the stomach is termed the lesser curvature, whereas the left convex edge is called the greater curvature. The peritoneal reflections, connecting the lesser curvature to the liver, form the lesser omentum, also called the gastrohepatic ligament. It contains branches of the left and right gastric arteries. Peritoneal reflections on the greater curvature side form the greater omentum and are subdivided by

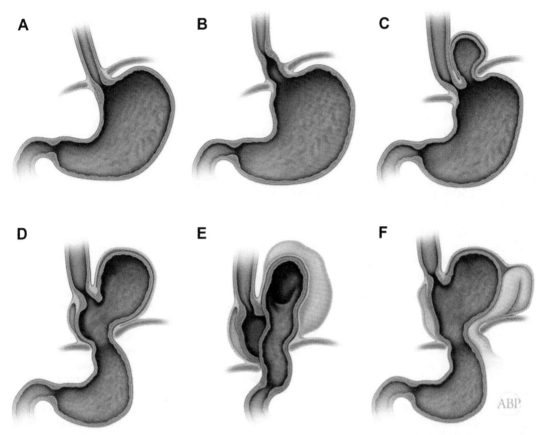

Fig. 2. Types of paraesophageal hernias. (*A*) Normal anatomy of the GEJ. (*B*) Type I (sliding) hiatal hernia. (*C*) Type II paraesophageal hernia. The GEJ is retained at the hiatus and fundus has herniated into the mediastinum through a localized defect at the phrenoesophageal membrane, with formation of peritoneal hernia sac. (*D*) Type III paraesophageal hernia (herniation of the GEJ and various degrees of the gastric fundus and the body into posterior mediastinum, with formation of the peritoneal hernia sac). (*E*) Type III paraesophageal hernia with totally intrathoracic stomach. (*F*) Type IV paraesophageal hernia with herniation of the other intraabdominal organs in addition to the GEJ and various degrees of the gastric fundus and the body with formation of the hernia sac.

the site of the attachment into gastrophrenic, gastrosplenic, and gastrocolic ligaments. They contain both right and left gastroepiploic branches from the pancreaticoduodenal and the splenic arteries that form an arch along the antrum and the body of the stomach about a centimeter lateral to the stomach wall. The fundus is directly supplied by the branches of the short gastric vessels.

DIAPHRAGM

The diaphragm is a complex flat dome-shaped fibromuscular structure that separates the chest from the abdomen. It has a central fibrous tendon and muscular fibers peripherally, attaching to the lumbar vertebrae in the back, lower 6 ribs on both sides, and xyphoid process anteriorly. Contraction of the muscular fibers results in the vertical displacement of the fibrous center of the diaphragm, providing a major contribution to the respiratory cycle. Several important structures cross the diaphragm. The inferior vena cava enters the chest through the opening in the central tendon and is accompanied by small branches of right phrenic nerve. The aorta with the accompanying thoracic duct traverses the diaphragm through aortic hiatus between the diaphragmatic crura. The splanchnic nerves, sympathetic chains, hemiazygos vein, and internal thoracic artery travel through an additional minor opening in the diaphragm. The esophagus with both vagus nerves traverses the diaphragm through the esophageal hiatus.

THE ESOPHAGEAL HIATUS

The esophageal hiatus is a slit-like opening in the diaphragm that is formed by the thickened bundles of the right crus and has a reverse tear-drop shape. The undersurface of the diaphragm is covered by the thin endoabdominal fascia, which forms the phrenoesophageal ligament at the hiatus. This ligament is a fibrotic sheath of connective tissue that inserts onto the adventitia of the distal esophagus, the GEJ, as well as the intraabdominal esophagus (**Fig. 1**B). Thus, the GEJ is usually located below the esophageal hiatus and is secured in position by the phrenoesophageal ligament.[3,4]

THE LOWER ESOPHAGEAL SPHINCTER AND ANATOMIC ANTIREFLUX SYSTEM

The thickening of the circular layer of the distal esophagus above the GEJ is called the lower esophageal sphincter (LES). The LES usually measures 2.5 to 4.5 cm in length, with the upper part lying within the hiatus and the lower part in the abdomen. The LES serves as a first component of the antireflux mechanism. Although not a true anatomic sphincter, it is defined as a high-pressure zone by manometry and is tonically contracted, providing a pressure gradient between the esophagus and the stomach. The short intraabdominal segment of the distal esophagus is exposed to the positive intraabdominal pressure and serves as an additional pressure barrier, aiding the LES in its antireflux function. The crura of the esophageal hiatus are another component, exerting lateral pinching of the distal esophagus, or the so-called pinchcock effect. In deep inspiration, pressure increases due to crural contraction when transdiaphragmatic pressure gradient also increases, preventing gastroesophageal reflux.[5–7] The third component of the antireflux mechanism is the angle of His, a flap valve comprising of the fundus, draping along the left side of the abdominal esophagus at an acute angle, which is held in place by the phrenoesophageal ligament.[8] The final physiologic mechanism for controlling reflux is the esophageal peristalsis. Mechanical and chemical receptors in the distal esophagus mediate esophageal clearance of intraluminal contents. Poor esophageal motility, in combination with acid reflux, may lead to esophagitis, which could further impair the function and the tone of the LES.[9]

PATHOPHYSIOLOGY OF HIATAL HERNIA DEVELOPMENT

Hiatal hernia occurs when a portion of the gastric cardia prolapses into the posterior mediastinum through the esophageal hiatus. This leads to misalignment of the LES and the crura, thus disrupting the protective anatomic defense mechanisms. Proximal migration of the LES transposes it into the negative pressure environment of the chest, diminishing the pressure gradient at the GEJ and obliterating the flap valve function of the angle of His. Moreover, lateral traction by the stretched phrenoesophageal membrane further compromises the LES function. Misalignment of the LES and the crura leads to pressure application on a funnel-like cardia, which tends to direct intragastric contents into the esophagus with the increase of intraabdominal pressure, promoting gastroesophageal reflux.[1]

The transdiaphragmatic pressure gradient, formed by the negative intrathoracic pressure (due to elastic recoil of the lung) and the positive intraabdominal pressure (due to the tonic contraction of the abdominal wall muscles), exerts a constant upward push on the GEJ. The deglutition process is associated with foreshortening of the esophagus. These, in addition to large-volume meals, distend the gastric fundus and lead to stretching and weakening the LES, an effect similar to that at the neck of an inflated balloon. Additional stressors on the phrenoesophageal ligament are associated with increased intraabdominal pressure, such as obesity, constipation, urinary obstruction, chronic obstructive pulmonary disease with chronic cough, and job-related heavy exertion. Restrictive lung disease may heighten the transdiaphragmatic pressure gradient owing to increased negative intrathoracic pressures. Impaired connective tissue integrity may also play a role in developing a paraesophageal hernia. Accordingly, paraesophageal hernias frequently present in elderly patients with comorbidities and degenerative diseases. It may also be associated with familial clustering, suggesting that genetic factors may also be a causal factor.[1,10,11]

TYPES OF HIATAL HERNIAS

Hiatal hernias are classified into 4 types according to the degree of the intrathoracic prolapse of the GEJ and its relationship to the herniated stomach (**Fig. 2**).[1,12,13]

Type I hiatal hernia is the most common type and represents more than 95% of all cases (see **Fig. 2**B).[1,13] It is probably the first step in the continuum of the progressive distention of the phrenoesophageal membrane and separation of the GEJ and crural diaphragm. It is frequently termed a sliding hernia. Contrary to the common misperception, it is not because it goes up and down but rather because it is a hernia that is formed by the wall of the organ itself, without a hernia sac.

Type II paraesophageal hernias form due to a local defect of the phrenoesophageal membrane, usually in the left posterior aspect. A true hernia sac forms through this defect, with intrathoracic herniation of the gastric fundus. The GEJ in a true type II hernia is below the hiatus, likely held in place by residual intact portion of the phrenoesophageal ligament (see **Fig. 2**C). For this reason, many of these patients may not suffer from GERD as the reflux barrier is still mostly intact. These hernias are quite infrequent.

Type III paraesophageal hernia is the most common type of paraesophageal hernias, and represent the continuous stretching of the phrenoesophageal ligament with increasing hiatal dilation and formation of the peritoneal hernia sac. The GEJ, in addition to part or all of the gastric fundus and body, migrate up (see **Fig. 2**D). In an extreme case, a patient may develop a totally intrathoracic stomach. As the size of the hernia sac continues to enlarge with relative fixation of the terminal esophagus to the prevertebral fascia, the greater curvature slides up, flipping over in the form of both organoaxial and mesoaxial rotation. This results in a twisted upside-down stomach in which the pylorus may be higher than the GEJ and the greater curvature is to the right of the esophagus (see **Fig. 2**E).

Type IV paraesophageal hernias are extreme forms of this condition in which, in addition to the majority of the stomach, other organs, such as the omentum, transverse colon, small intestines, spleen, liver, and even retroperitoneal structures (including the pancreas) can herniate (see **Fig. 2**F).

RECURRENT PARAESOPHAGEAL HERNIAS

Recurrent paraesophageal hernias represent a particularly challenging situation because anatomic derangements occur in the previously

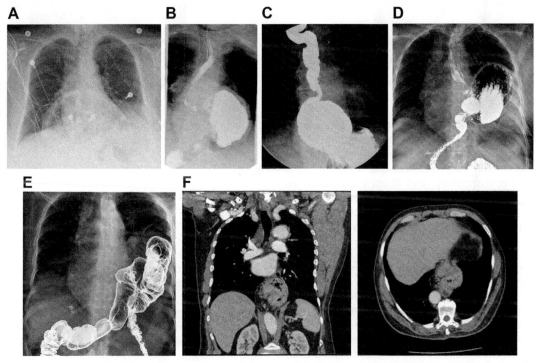

Fig. 3. Radiologic evaluation of paraesophageal hernias. (*A*) Chest radiograph demonstrating retrocardiac lucency, consistent with paraesophageal hernia. (*B*) Esophagram, demonstrating type II paraesophageal hernia. Please note normal position of the GEJ. (*C*) Esophagram, demonstrating type III paraesophageal hernia. (*D*) Esophagram, demonstrating type III paraesophageal hernia with totally intrathoracic stomach. (*E*) Barium enema, demonstrating type IV paraesophageal hernia with intrathoracic colon (coronal reconstruction [*left*] and axial image [*right*]). (*F*) Computed tomography (CT) demonstrating type III paraesophageal hernia. (*G*) CT demonstrating type IV paraesophageal hernia, with totally intrathoracic stomach and colon (coronal reconstruction [*left*] and axial image [*right*]). (*H*) CT, demonstrating type IV paraesophageal hernia with a large posterior component and herniated retroperitoneum and pancreatic tail. (*I*) Esophagram, demonstrating recurrent paraesophageal hernia with posterior crural disruption, leading to small bowel herniation but normal position of the GEJ (gastric faze, showing normal intraabdominal position of the stomach [*left*] and intestinal faze, demonstrating transhiatal herniation of the small bowel [*right*]). (*J*) Paraconduit hernia in a patient after previous minimally invasive esophagectomy.

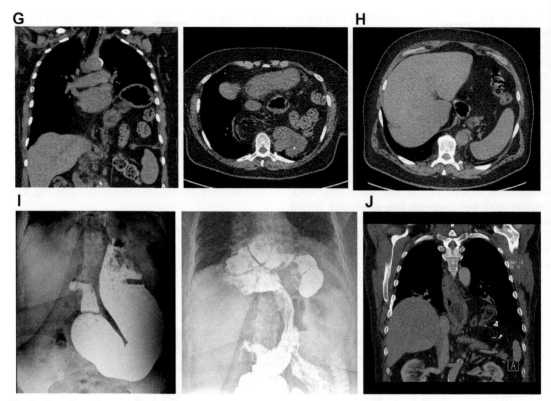

Fig. 3. (*continued*)

operated field with loss of the normal tissue planes due to scarring. A clear understanding of the anatomic relationship requires extensive preoperative workup with functional and cross-sectional imaging, manometry, and direct visualization via endoscopy (**Fig. 3**F). Review of the previous operative record is mandatory for extrapolation of the anatomic relationships after a previous surgical procedure.

PARACONDUIT POSTESOPHAGECTOMY HIATAL HERNIAS

After esophagectomy, a neoesophageal conduit (tubularized stomach or colon) traverses the diaphragm. This creates a potential defect between the conduit and the edges of the hiatus, potentially leading to herniation of abdominal contents into the chest. These hernias can form on any side of the conduit, although it is the left posterior aspect of the hiatus that is more commonly herniated (**Fig. 3**J). Because these hernias have no hernia sac and the peritoneal cavity communicates directly with the pleural space, large segments of small and large intestines pass through the hiatus and translocate into the chest.[14,15] Laparoscopic surgery is known to be associated with less fibrosis and fewer adhesions than traditional open procedures. The increasing adoption of minimally invasive

techniques esophagectomy has likely led to an increase in the incidence of paraconduit hernias.

RADIOLOGICAL ANATOMY

Imaging studies are an important step in preoperative patient evaluation. Occasionally, the presence of a paraesophageal hernia can be suspected on a chest radiograph, with demonstration of retrocardiac air-fluid level or lucency (**Fig. 3**A). An esophagram with fluoroscopy allows a thorough assessment of the anatomy, the configuration of the gastrointestinal tract, and the swallowing function (**Fig. 3**B–D, I). Computed tomography provides further assessment of the size of the hernia and hiatal defect; configuration of the stomach; size and content of the hernia sac, with the degree of the adjacent structures compression; and involvement of the other intraabdominal organs (**Fig. 3**F–H, J).[16–18] Additional studies might be indicated to assess the involvement of other organs (**Fig. 3**E).

ENDOSCOPIC ANATOMY

Endoscopy is mandatory in evaluation of all paraesophageal hernias before repair. Anatomic evaluation of the paraesophageal hernias during endoscopy includes assessment of the hernia size, status of the LES, and presence of complications, such as strictures, Barret esophagus, or even tumors.[19] The retroflexion endoscopic view provides important observation into the type and grading of the GEJ.[8] In patients with paraesophageal hernias, a Hill type IV junction is present, with the extrinsic impression of the dilated hiatal opening along with the various degree of herniated stomach.

Measurement of the paraesophageal hernia is accomplished by subtraction of the distance from the incisors to the Z-line from that of the incisors to the hiatus. Owing to distention of the stomach by the insufflated air, most of the organ pops back into the subdiaphragmatic position. In cases of large paraesophageal hernias with most of the intrathoracic stomach in organoaxial or mesoaxial rotation, it is sometimes difficult to find the hiatus and the passage into the subdiaphragmatic stomach. Any attempt at accurate length measurement in these cases can be unreliable (**Fig. 4**A-C).

SURGICAL ANATOMY

Paraesophageal hernias may be approached from the abdomen or the chest. The most common modality is undoubtedly laparoscopic. However, in certain cases, an open laparotomy may be necessary. In case of multiple recurrences or a hostile abdomen from previous surgeries, the thoracic approach may be preferred. The surgeons must therefore familiarize themselves with the different appearance of the anatomy through every approach.

ANATOMIC EXPOSURE WITH LAPAROTOMY

An open hiatal hernia abdominal repair is usually performed through an upper midline laparotomy with extension above the xyphoid process. Effective elevation of the costal margin is required for adequate exposure. The left lobe of the liver covers the hiatus and is mobilized by dividing the left triangular ligament and retracting it to the right. This maneuver exposes both the central tendon and the esophageal hiatus of the diaphragm.

The hiatus is usually obviously dilated. The lesser omentum is stretched over the right crus and follows the lesser curvature into the mediastinum. After manual reduction of the stomach, the previously stretched phrenoesophageal membrane appears floppy after hernia reduction. It is grasped and opened, allowing visualization and circumferential mobilization of the esophagus. This is followed by division of the phrenoesophageal membrane and dissection of the sac.[20,21]

The esophagus is retracted anteriorly and to the left, exposing the posterior hiatus. The crura are approximated, leaving at least a 1-cm space between the esophageal wall and the edge of the hiatus. An antireflux procedure of choice is then performed before conclusion of the repair.[22]

TRANSTHORACIC ANATOMY

Transthoracic anatomy is usually accomplished through the left chest. Video-assisted thoracoscopic surgery (VATS) modification has not gained wide adoption and there are only limited reports of VATS.[23,24] Robotic transabdominal modification of Belsey repair technique has also been described.[25]

The patient is positioned in the right lateral decubitus position and a left posterolateral thoracotomy is performed in seventh or eighth intercostal space. The inferior pulmonary ligament is divided and the lung is retracted superiorly. The descending aorta is visible in the field and the esophagus with the paraesophageal hernia is identified immediately anterior and medial to it. The left atrium is located anteriorly to the hernia sac. Opening of the hernia sac allows dissection of the crura. The esophagus is mobilized sufficiently to allow tension-free repair.

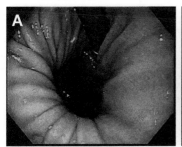 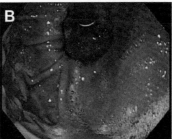 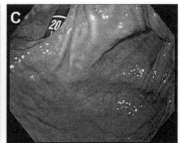

Fig. 4. Endoscopic anatomy of paraesophageal hernias. (*A*) Endoscopy, demonstrating type II paraesophageal hernia on the retroflexion view. Please note normal position of the GEJ and herniation of the fundus. (*B*) Endoscopy, demonstrating type III paraesophageal hernia. (*C*) Endoscopy, demonstrating, type III paraesophageal hernia, with totally intrathoracic stomach. Please note location of gastric outlet next to GEJ due to organoaxial and mesoaxial rotation.

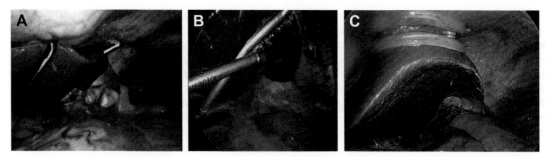

Fig. 5. Liver retractors. (*A*) Nathanson liver retractor. (*B*) Flexible liver retractor. (*C*) LiVac retractor. (*Courtesy of* [*A*] Dr. Warner W. Wang, MD, Marietta, OH; and [*C*] Dr. Philip Gan, Livac Pty Ltd, Warrnambool, Australia.)

MINIMALLY INVASIVE, LAPAROSCOPIC ANATOMY

The laparoscopic approach has enjoyed wide acceptance owing to the benefits associated with minimally invasive surgery.[22,26] Laparoscopy, either traditional or robotically enhanced, allows a significant advantage in visualization and magnification of the target anatomy, facilitating dissection and repair. With the camera usually placed in the left epigastric area, the viewing trajectory is right along the esophagus, clearly depicting the hiatus, gastroesophageal junction, esophagus, and structures of the posterior mediastinum.[27–32]

Exposure of the hiatus requires elevation of the left lobe of the liver. Either a Nathanson retractor, placed through the subxyphoid area, or a flexible retractor, placed through right flank port, is used for these purposes (**Fig. 5**A, B).[13,33,34] The LiVac vacuum liver retractor (Livac Pty Ltd, Warrnambool, Australia) has recently been introduced into clinical practice for this purpose (**Fig. 5**C). Obese patients, especially men, may have a significantly enlarged and fragile left lobe of the liver due to a fatty liver and this is prone to injury and bleeding. This may complicate exposure of the relevant anatomy. Women, in contrast, more often have a thin and floppy left lobe of the liver, reaching over the spleen, which may require reapplication of the retractor throughout the procedure.

Again, the hiatus is dilated and is oval to round in shape (**Fig. 6**A). The phrenoesophageal membrane is stretched and is bulging into the mediastinum, augmented by positive intraabdominal pressure of the pneumoperitoneum. The stomach, unless incarcerated by adhesions, usually freely retracts into the abdomen. Occasionally, there is a posterior crural diastasis, accompanied by significant posterior component of the hernia sac. In such scenario, a large volume of the retroperitoneal fat is prolapsed into the chest in the form of a mediastinal lipoma. This can involve prolapse of the retroperitoneal organs (pancreas and spleen) causing the type IV hernia.

The esophagus is mobilized high into the mediastinum with a coaxial close-up view of camera visualization. Mobilization starts with opening of the phrenoesophageal membrane and hernia sac, usually anteriorly, which allows entrance in to the mediastinal tissue.[13,28,35] The CO2 creates a foamy appearance of the loose connective tissue of the mediastinum, with easy identification of any vessels (**Fig. 6**B). With good visualization, mobilization of the thoracic esophagus to the subcarinal area is possible. At this point, the surgeon should identify the membranous airway and minimize

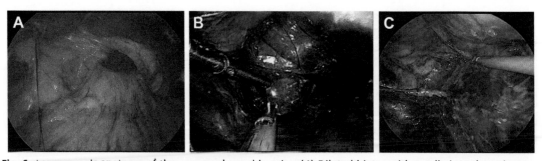

Fig. 6. Laparoscopic anatomy of the paraesophageal hernias. (*A*) Dilated hiatus with totally intrathoracic stomach. Greater curvature is visible in the hernia sac and the greater omentum draping over the hiatus. (*B*) Foamy appearance of the mediastinal tissue signifies the correct plane of dissection. (*C*) Subcarinal lymph node pocket and thoracic duct exposed along the thoracic aorta are visible during the dissection.

use of cautery to avoid an airway injury (**Fig. 6**C). Posteriorly, the esophagus is mobilized from the aorta, and aortoesophageal branches are controlled. Laterally, the pleural membranes can be identified and protected from injury. Premature pleural injury results in the collapse of the mediastinal space, complicating the dissection and anatomic exposure. The thoracic duct runs on the right posterior aspect of the aorta and its injury is uncommon (**Fig. 6**C). However, due to the variability of its course, a high index of suspicion is mandatory and, if there is concern regarding possible injury, prophylactic ligation may be advised.

SUMMARY

Paraesophageal hernias represent a complex surgical problem. Surgeons tackling this disease should become familiar with the complex anatomic relationships in this condition. Indeed, the tenets of a successful and durable repair of this disease require reconstruction of the normal anatomy, including the diaphragmatic hiatus and the abdominal esophagus. Careful identification and avoidance of the vagus nerves is essential. Comprehensive understanding of the anatomy of the diaphragm, esophagus, and stomach will allow the surgeon to be comfortable in performing this operation through the abdomen or the chest.

ACKNOWLEDGEMENT

This research was funded in part through the NIH/NCI Cancer Center Support Grant P30 CA006927.

REFERENCES

1. Jobe BA, Hunter JG, Watson DI. Esophagus and diaphragmatic hernia. In: Brunicardi FC, Andersen DK, Billiar TR, et al, editors. Schwartz's principles of surgery. 10th edition. New York: McGraw-Hill Education; 2014.

2. Zhang X, Patil D, Odze RD, et al. The microscopic anatomy of the esophagus including the individual layers, specialized tissues, and unique components and their responses to injury. Ann N Y Acad Sci 2018;1434(1):304–18.

3. Botros KG, El-Ayat AA, El-Naggar MM, et al. The development of the human phreno-oesophageal membrane. Acta Anat (Basel) 1983;115(1):23–30.

4. Eliska O. Phreno-oesophageal membrane and its role in the development of hiatal hernia. Acta Anat (Basel) 1973;86(1):137–50.

5. Mittal RK, Zifan A, Kumar D, et al. Functional morphology of the lower esophageal sphincter and crural diaphragm determined by three-dimensional high-resolution esophago-gastric junction pressure profile and CT imaging. Am J Physiol Gastrointest Liver Physiol 2017;313(3):G212–9.

6. Costa MM, Pires-Neto MA. Anatomical investigation of the esophageal and aortic hiatuses: physiologic, clinical and surgical considerations. Anat Sci Int 2004;79(1):21–31.

7. Kahrilas PJ, Lin S, Chen J, et al. The effect of hiatus hernia on gastro-oesophageal junction pressure. Gut 1999;44(4):476–82.

8. Hill LD, Kozarek RA, Kraemer SJ, et al. The gastroesophageal flap valve: in vitro and in vivo observations. Gastrointest Endosc 1996;44(5):541–7.

9. Iwakiri K. The role of excessive esophageal acid exposure in patients with gastroesophageal reflux disease. Clin J Gastroenterol 2009;2(6):371–9.

10. Bohmer AC, Schumacher J. Insights into the genetics of gastroesophageal reflux disease (GERD) and GERD-related disorders. Neurogastroenterol Motil 2017;29(2). https://doi.org/10.1111/nmo.13017.

11. Herbella FA, Patti MG. Gastroesophageal reflux disease: from pathophysiology to treatment. World J Gastroenterol 2010;16(30):3745–9.

12. Hagarty G. A classification of esophageal hiatus hernia with special reference to sliding hernia. Am J Roentgenol Radium Ther Nucl Med 1960;84:1056–60.

13. Oleynikov D, Jolley JM. Paraesophageal hernia. Surg Clin North Am 2015;95(3):555–65.

14. Kent MS, Luketich JD, Tsai W, et al. Revisional surgery after esophagectomy: an analysis of 43 patients. Ann Thorac Surg 2008;86(3):975–83 [discussion: 967–74].

15. Gust L, Nafteux P, Allemann P, et al. Hiatal hernia after oesophagectomy: a large European survey. Eur J Cardiothorac Surg 2019;55(6):1104–12.

16. Tsunoda S, Jamieson GG, Devitt PG, et al. Early reoperation after laparoscopic fundoplication: the importance of routine postoperative contrast studies. World J Surg 2010;34(1):79–84.

17. Burdan F, Rozylo-Kalinowska I, Szumilo J, et al. Anatomical classification of the shape and topography of the stomach. Surg Radiol Anat 2012;34(2):171–8.

18. Abbas AE. The management of gastroesophageal reflux disease. In: Cameron JL, Cameron AM, editors. Current surgical therapy. 12th edition. Philadelphia: Elsevier Health Sciences; 2016. p. 10–9.

19. Tatum JM, Samakar K, Bowdish ME, et al. Videoesophagography versus endoscopy for prediction of intraoperative hiatal hernia size. Am Surg 2018;84(3):387–91.

20. Johnson AB, Oddsdottir M, Hunter JG. Laparoscopic Collis gastroplasty and Nissen fundoplication. A new technique for the management of esophageal foreshortening. Surg Endosc 1998;12(8):1055–60.

21. Terry ML, Vernon A, Hunter JG. Stapled-wedge Collis gastroplasty for the shortened esophagus. Am J Surg 2004;188(2):195–9.

22. Goldberg MB, Abbas AE, Smith MS, et al. Minimally invasive fundoplication is safe and effective in patients with severe esophageal hypomotility. Innovations (Phila) 2016;11(6):396–9.

23. Nguyen NT, Schauer PR, Hutson W, et al. Preliminary results of thoracoscopic Belsey Mark IV antireflux procedure. Surg Laparosc Endosc 1998;8(3):185–8.

24. Molena D, Mungo B, Stem M, et al. Novel combined VATS/laparoscopic approach for giant and complicated paraesophageal hernia repair: description of technique and early results. Surg Endosc 2015; 29(1):185–91.

25. Gharagozloo F, Atiquzzaman B, Tempesta B, et al. Long-term results of robotic modified Belsey (gastroesophageal valvuloplasty) fundoplication. Surg Technol Int 2018;34:121–7.

26. Bakhos CT, Fabian T, Oyasiji TO, et al. Impact of the surgical technique on pulmonary morbidity after esophagectomy. Ann Thorac Surg 2012;93(1): 221–6 [discussion: 226–7].

27. Terry M, Smith CD, Branum GD, et al. Outcomes of laparoscopic fundoplication for gastroesophageal reflux disease and paraesophageal hernia. Surg Endosc 2001;15(7):691–9.

28. Luketich JD, Nason KS, Christie NA, et al. Outcomes after a decade of laparoscopic giant paraesophageal hernia repair. J Thorac Cardiovasc Surg 2010; 139(2):395–404, 404.e1.

29. Lerut T, Deschamps C. Techniques for repair of paraesophageal hiatal hernia. In: Sugarbaker DJ, Bueno R, Colson YL, et al, editors. Adult chest surgery. 2nd edition. New York: McGraw-Hill Education; 2015.

30. Sarkaria IS, Latif MJ, Bianco VJ, et al. Early operative outcomes and learning curve of robotic assisted giant paraesophageal hernia repair. Int J Med Robot 2017;13(1). https://doi.org/10.1002/rcs.1730.

31. Vasudevan V, Reusche R, Nelson E, et al. Robotic paraesophageal hernia repair: a single-center experience and systematic review. J Robot Surg 2018; 12(1):81–6.

32. Mertens AC, Tolboom RC, Zavrtanik H, et al. Morbidity and mortality in complex robot-assisted hiatal hernia surgery: 7-year experience in a high-volume center. Surg Endosc 2019;33(7):2152–61.

33. Petrov R, Bakhos C, Abbas A. Robotic-assisted minimally invasive esophagectomy. In: Kudsi Y, Carbonell A, Yiengpruksawan A, et al, editors. Atlas of robotic surgery. Woodbury (CT): Cine-Med; 2018. p. 106–53.

34. Nason KS, Luketich JD, Witteman BP, et al. The laparoscopic approach to paraesophageal hernia repair. J Gastrointest Surg 2012;16(2):417–26.

35. Petrov R, Bakhos C, Abbas A. Robotic esophagectomy. In: Tsuda S, Kudsi OY, editors. Robotic-assisted minimally invasive surgery. Cham (Switzerland): Springer Nature; 2019. p. 277–93.

Surgical Techniques for Robotically-Assisted Laparoscopic Paraesophageal Hernia Repair

Chigozirim N. Ekeke, MD, Matthew Vercauteren, PA-C,
Nicholas Baker, MD*, Inderpal Sarkaria, MD

KEYWORDS

- Robotic-assisted laparoscopic paraesophageal hernia repair • Giant paraesophageal hernia
- Robotic-surgery

KEY POINTS

- For a successful robotic-assisted giant paraesophageal hernia repair, reduce the stomach and the associated intrathoracic contents including the hernia sac with extensive mediastinal dissection.
- For a successful robotic-assisted giant paraesophageal hernia repair, reestablish adequate intraabdominal esophageal length and perform a Collis gastroplasty if needed.
- For a successful robotic-assisted giant paraesophageal hernia repair, perform a diaphragmatic defect closure (with or without mesh).
- For a successful robotic-assisted giant paraesophageal hernia repair, establish anti reflux barrier (or gastropexy, if needed).

 Video content accompanies this article at http://www.thoracic.theclinics.com.

INTRODUCTION

Minimally invasive surgery has been introduced as a safe approach for repairing giant paraesophageal hernias (GPEH), without the rates of morbidity and mortality associated with an open approach (Video 1).[1–4] Given existing studies on the feasibility of minimally invasive approach to GPEH repair, the laparoscopic approach remains at the forefront in managing this disease process. Decreases in blood loss, intraoperative complications, and length of stay have been attributed to the minimally invasive approach, despite an increase in comorbidity in the patient population.[2,3]

As of late, the robotic approach to GPEH has become increasingly popular and yields technically superior procedural aspects in comparison to the conventional laparoscopic approach, mainly in improved stable optics, degrees of freedom of motion, improved 3-dimensional high-definition view, intuitive movements, tremor filtering, and the ability to self-first assist.[5,6] Despite these advantages, the learning curve must be considered given the technical demands of these procedures, requiring extensive adhesiolysis, hernia sac dissection, and esophageal mobilization within the mediastinum, where maintaining visualization for extended periods of time can be challenging.[5]

Disclosure Statement: The authors have nothing to disclose.
Department of Cardiothoracic Surgery, University of Pittsburgh Medical Center, 9100 Babcock Boulevard, Pittsburgh, PA 15237, USA
* Corresponding author.
E-mail address: bakern2@upmc.edu

Data showing comparisons between robotic approaches and open and laparoscopic remain largely scarce. Gehrig and colleagues[7,8] conducted a case control study displaying no differences in operative times in either approach, but the intraoperative and postoperative complication rates were lower for robotic and laparoscopic, 16.7% and 17.6%, respectively, when compared with the open approach (58%).

We have conducted a retrospective study assessing early outcomes in patients presenting with symptomatic GPEHs who underwent robotic-assisted GPEH repair over a 3-year period. The median age was 62 years and 63% of the patients (n = 15) underwent fundoplication and 37% (n = 9) for gastropexy. The median operative time was 277 minutes and decreased steadily over the experience. There were no intraoperative complications or surgical mortality, and there were no complaints of dysphagia in the early postoperative period.[6]

PREOPERATIVE ASSESSMENT

A full history and physical examination must be performed and the surgeon must elicit specific symptoms (regurgitation, heartburn, waterbrash), aspiration, cough, abdominal pain, chest discomfort, and dysphagia. A barium esophagram is performed to assess esophageal motility, reflux, and severity of herniation and anatomic relationship between stomach, gastroesophageal junction, and diaphragmatic hiatus. A barium esophagram allows the surgeon to identify the anatomic contours of alimentary tract and presence of volvulus or endoluminal disease. Laboratory studies include hemoglobin and hematocrit to assess for anemia. A computed tomography scan is not routinely performed unless there is high suspicion for other pathology or to identify type IV GPEH. Manometry studies are not performed on every patient, because these studies have an inherent risk of placement difficulty, poor accuracy, and even esophageal perforation. Preoperative and intraoperative endoscopy should be performed to assess stomach viability, gastroesophageal junction location, occult malignancy, Barrett's esophagus, diverticular disease, or other pathology. We advocate that the endoscopic evaluation is performed by the surgeon, at the very least, on the day of surgery.

Relative contraindications include an inability to tolerate general anesthesia, severe cardiopulmonary dysfunction, or an uncontrolled hematologic disorder. Patient age, the size of the hernia, and previous abdominal surgeries are not contraindications. When possible, a period of resuscitation is advisable before surgery to correct physiologic and laboratory derangements.

TECHNIQUE

The patient is placed in the supine position, followed by general anesthesia induction and subsequent orotracheal intubation. An arterial line is placed for hemodynamic monitoring. Careful endoscopic evaluation with minimal air insufflation is conducted by the surgeon. Excessive air insufflation would present technical challenges during laparoscopic visualization and robotic assistance. In obstructed patients, excessive air may cause gastric dilation, vagal stimulation, and possibly severe hemodynamic instability. During endoscopic assessment, the surgeon should thoroughly inspect the esophagus to rule out occult malignancy, confirm the level of the gastroesophageal junction, and decompress the stomach. A footboard is placed to support reverse Trendelenburg positioning. We prefer keeping both arms out at 45°, but the left arm can be tucked at the surgeon's discretion. A liver retractor (DiamondFlex, Snowden Pencer, Vernon Hills, IL) is used; thus, the patient is placed to the right of the operating table. The operating table is positioned 90° and the robotic arms and cart (DaVinci Si, Intuitive Surgical, Sunnyvale, CA) are brought in over the midline and into position to allow entry and exit (**Fig. 1**).

The procedure is performed using 6 ports. Appropriate port placement is pivotal to a successful operation owing to the extensive mediastinal dissection necessary to reduce the hernia contents, excise the hernia sac, and adequately mobilize the esophagus. To facilitate this goal, the midline from the xiphoid to the level of the umbilicus is marked and divided in thirds. A camera incision is marked just left of the midline in the midabdomen, approximately half the distance from the xiphoid to the umbilicus. A left lateral subcostal 8-mm incision is marked for using the robotic atraumatic grasper for assistance. This may be a 5-mm incision on less recent versions of the robotic platform (DaVinci Si Platform, Intuitive Surgical, Sunnyvale, CA). Subsequently, left midclavicular 8-mm incision is marked at the left epigastrium, one fingerbreadth below the ribs. This port is used as the robotic right hand and for the robotic ultrasonic shears. An additional 8-mm right midclavicular port is marked at the epigastrium for bipolar fenestrated forceps (robotic left hand). This port is kept close to the midline to minimize the instrument angulation between the shaft and right crural pillar during transhiatal intrathoracic dissection. The liver retractor is inserted through a right lateral 5-mm subcostal

Room setup and patient positioning

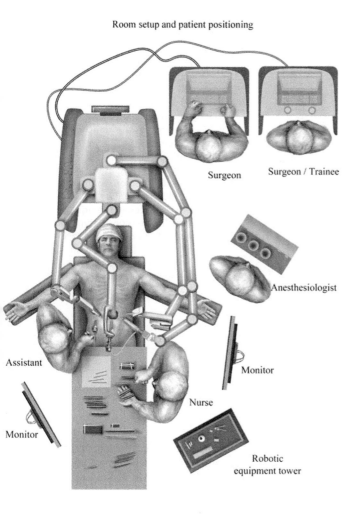

Surgeon

Surgeon / Trainee

Anesthesiologist

Assistant

Monitor

Nurse

Monitor

Robotic
equipment tower

Fig. 1. Operating room set up for robotically assisted GPEH repair. (*From* Karush J, Sarkaria IS. Robotic-assisted giant paraesophageal hernia repair and Nissen fundoplication. Oper Tech Thorac Cardiovasc Surg. 2013;18(3):205; with permission.)

port. A 12-mm port is placed at the level of the right periumbilical plane. Of note, we deem it critical to maintain at least an 8- to 10-cm distance between robotic ports to minimize collisions, and all ports are placed under visualization. More recent versions of the robotic platforms (DaVinci Xi Platform, Intuitive Surgical) allow closer placement of these ports without undue arm collisions, and the ability to advance the care independently of bed position. For optimal peritoneal distension and visualization, 15 mm Hg of CO_2 insufflation is provided. Port placements are summarized in **Fig. 2**.

HERNIA SAC REDUCTION

The patient is placed in reverse Trendelenburg to assist with adequate visualization of the hiatus. It is important to remember, many patients receive 1 L of polyethylene glycol electrolyte solution as bowel preparation and are prone to fluid shifts resulting in hemodynamic changes during

positional changes at the beginning of the case. After reverse Trendelenburg is slowly achieved, we proceed to reduce the hernia contents (ie, omental fat, bowel) to achieve optimal visualization of the hiatus (**Fig. 3**). Sac reduction is achieved by grasping the hernia sac at 12 o'clock and atraumatically everting the hernia sac (**Fig. 4**). Using careful dissection, the layers of the weakened phrenoesophageal ligament and peritoneal reflection are divided with care to avoid injury to the widened anterior aspect of the crural pillars. After entering the posterior mediastinum, the surgeon can use the robotic ultrasonic shears to divide this largely areolar plane. Visualizing the arealor attachments is critical during this portion of the case, because it ensures that the surgeon is safely visualizing the posterior mediastinal boundaries and critical contents (bilateral pleurae, pericardium, esophagus, aorta, vertebrae, hemi-azygous vein, thoracic duct, pulmonary veins, and vagal nerves). During the sac dissection, the surgeon must visualize the pleural reflection to avoid causing an

Port placement

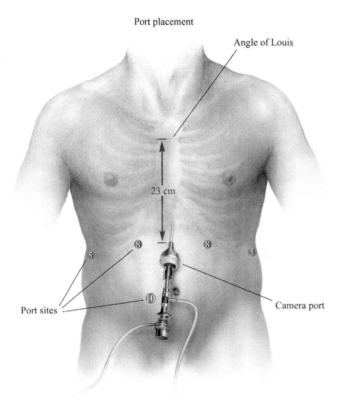

Angle of Louis

23 cm

Port sites

Camera port

Fig. 2. Port placement. An 8-mm robotic trocar is placed at the left lateral costal margin, in which a 5-mm atraumatic grasper is used as the robotic assistant. Second, a left 8-mm port for the harmonic device is placed at the midclavicular line, 1 to 2 cm below the costal margin. Third, a 5-mm port is placed in the right lateral subcostal margin for the liver retractor and a robotic 8-mm trocar is placed in the right upper quadrant at the level of the midclavicular region, for the bipolar fenestrated grasper. Last, a 12-mm assistant port is placed in the right periumbilical umbilical region. (*From* Karush J, Sarkaria IS. Robotic-assisted giant paraesophageal hernia repair and Nissen fundoplication. Oper Tech Thorac Cardiovasc Surg. 2013;18(3):206; with permission.)

iatrogenic pneumothorax. If the pleural reflection is violated, the surgeon and anesthesiologist must communicate because a tension pneumothorax may quickly result in hemodynamic instability. Simply ceasing gas insufflation while evacuating the pneumothorax through the pleural defect with a laparoscopic suction device is the most effective immediate maneuver. Many patients tolerate these small rents without issue, despite the loss of visualization that may occur with collapse of the pleura into the mediastinal space. If this maneuver fails, insertion of a small bore pigtail and/or reducing abdominal CO_2 insufflation may lessen the hemodynamic dysfunction. Extensive dissection is performed until the sac is reduced, with care to avoid injuring the anterior and posterior vagus nerve. Mediastinal dissection is continued until the inferior pulmonary veins are visualized, at minimum (**Fig. 5**).

After successfully reducing the sac from the mediastinum, the sac must be dissected off the crural pillars bilaterally. While separating the sac from the crura, care must be taken to avoid damaging the peritoneal lining overlying the crura and exposing the muscle beneath. If the peritoneal lining is stripped from the underlying muscle, the integrity of the sutured crural reapproximation and closure may be at higher risk for dehiscence.

We believe extensive mediastinal mobilization and adequate sac reduction is critical to establishing a tension-free repair and decreasing the risk of recurrence.

ESOPHAGEAL LENGTH ASSESSMENT AND REESTABLISHING INTRAABDOMINAL ESOPHAGEAL LENGTH

After reducing the hernia stomach and its associated contents with crural preservation, the esophagus is further mobilized to the level of the inferior pulmonary veins or further cephalad. Again, care is taken to visualize and preserve the vagus nerves. Extensive mobilization allows for accurate assessment of esophageal length.

Upon completing esophageal mobilization, we proceed with mobilizing the gastric fundus by ligating the gastrosplenic attachments and short gastric arteries using ultrasonic energy. Care is taken to avoid traction injury to the spleen. The gastric attachments to the left crus are completely divided to optimize fundus mobilization, again, with care to preserve the peritoneal lining overlying the left crus. Following fundus mobilization, the gastric fat pad is mobilized medially off the stomach (**Fig. 6**) and distal

Initial exposure and hernia reduction

Dilated esophageal hiatus with peritoneal reflection in tact and extruding into thorax under pressure from abdominal insuflation

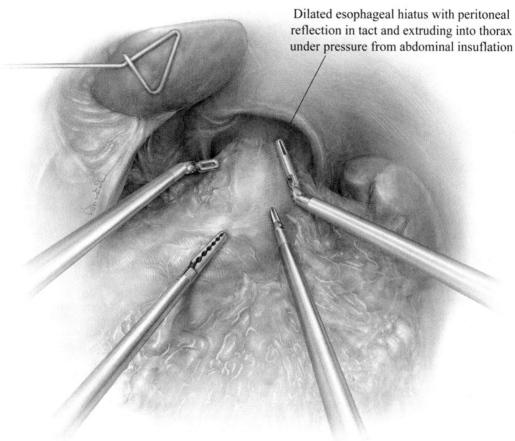

Fig. 3. The patient is in reverse Trendelenburg to use gravity in reducing the hernia's content. The remaining herniated contents are reduced from the mediastinum in the intraabdominal cavity with the use of robotic and bedside assistant ports. (*From* Karush J, Sarkaria IS. Robotic-assisted giant paraesophageal hernia repair and Nissen fundoplication. Oper Tech Thorac Cardiovasc Surg. 2013;18(3):207; with permission.)

esophagus to adequately and accurately visualize the gastroesophageal junction. Assessing the gastroesophageal junction allows for adequate intraabdominal length in the neutral resting position. At least 2.5 cm of intraabdominal esophagus is recommended to achieve a tension-free repair. Additional mediastinal mobilization may be performed if more than 2 cm of an intraabdominal esophagus is not achieved. In the event esophageal length is inadequate despite extensive mediastinal esophageal mobilization, an esophageal lengthening procedure is performed. Our preferred approach is a modified (wedge) Collis gastroplasty.

COLLIS GASTROPLASTY

A 54F bougie is inserted under direct visualization along the lesser curvature of the stomach to ensure safe gastric insertion. The right hand robotic working port is upsized to a 12-mm robotic stapler port. We use a robotic endostapler (45-mm EndoWrist Stapler with 3.5-mm blue staple loads) insert into this left subcostal robotic port (see **Fig. 2**). The first staple line is directly parallel to the line of the fundus and continued until the stapler closely approximates the bougie. The second staple line is carried horizontal to the axis of the esophagus and in tight apposition to the bougie. Care should be taken to avoid incorporating the esophageal body or vagus nerve into the stapler. Serial staple lines are performed in parallel with esophagus to complete a wedge resection of the stomach. The staple line establishes the new greater curve for the neoesophagus with the goal to obtain 2 to 3 cm of additional length.

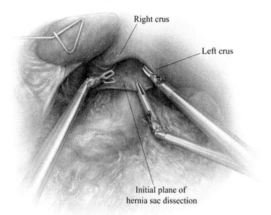

Right crus

Left crus

Initial plane of
hernia sac dissection

Fig. 4. After reducing the herniated contents, the hernial defect can be well-visualized. The hernia sac along is grasped at 12 o'clock and retracted inferiorly therefore, exposing the initial line of dissection between the sac and anterior crura. Sac dissection is initiated by incising the sac just below the anterior crura and developing a plane posterior to the pericardium, with attention to the peritoneal reflection. In most hernias, the areolar plane is mobilized with blunt dissection using the ultrasonic shears. This plane is largely avascular; therefore, there should be minimal blood loss during dissection. (*From* Karush J, Sarkaria IS. Robotic-assisted giant paraesophageal hernia repair and Nissen fundoplication. Oper Tech Thorac Cardiovasc Surg. 2013;18(3):208; with permission.)

HIATAL REPAIR

The hiatus is repaired in all patients. Care is taken to preserve the crural muscle fibers during mediastinal dissection to have adequate crural symphysis after closure. The robotic arm can be used to retract the crura laterally without grasping them during mediastinal dissection. To achieve a tension-free closure, additional dissection may be necessary if the crura are tethered by the phrenogastric or phrenosplenic ligament. Attention to identifying the pleural and peritoneal reflection is key to maintaining the integrity of both crural pillars. Inducing a left pneumothorax via a 5-mm intrathoracic port may provide significant laxity to the left hemidiaphragm and greatly aid in accomplishing a tension-free hiatal approximation. In this event, a pigtail catheter may be placed on the side of the pneumothorax after repair and removed at the surgeon's discretion.

The freely mobilized left and right crural pillars are approximated using 2 to 3 interrupted 0-polyester permanent braided suture, placed posteriorly. If there is significant space anteriorly, additional crural sutures are placed. The robotic assistant arm helps to retract the esophagus

superiorly and leftward, allowing for adequate exposure of the crura. Only the broad side of the retracting instrument should be used against the esophagus or stomach, especially while the bougie is in place, to avoid iatrogenic perforation. After closure, we evaluate the crura to ensure no excessive narrowing or impingement of the esophagus that would cause postoperative dysphagia.

Of note, bioprosthetic mesh or the use of pledget material can reinforce the crura or crural sutures in the event the pillars are severely denuded, or if there is concern for excessive crural tension. In our practice, the use of mesh is rare in primary cases.

ESTABLISHING AN ANTIREFLUX BARRIER

Owing to extensive esophageal dissection that would likely lead to significant gastroesophageal reflux, we typically create a new antireflux barrier. Surgeon preference, patient symptoms and preoperative physiologic testing and radiographic studies assessing esophageal motility dictate whether we perform a partial fundoplication or circumferential fundoplication (floppy Nissen).

NISSEN FUNDOPLICATION

The surgeon inserts a 54F bougie under visualization (**Figs. 7** and **8**). Use the atraumatic grasper in the 5-mm port to grasp the lateral of the staple line at the proximal fundus and pull through the retroesophageal window. The retractor in the robotic assistant arm port is able to retract the posterior aspect of the distal esophagus anteriorly and leftward, allowing passage of the proximal fundus through the retroesophageal window. If there is adequate fundus mobilization, the wrap will remain intact despite grasper release from the stomach, but further retrogastric mobilization is needed if this is not the case.

The graspers in the 8-mm L robotic arm port and the 5-mm robotic port contain the staple line from the Collis and lateral border of the short gastric arteries, respectively. A shoe-shine maneuver is performed after the wrap is pulled through the window. To secure the wrap, 2-0 polyester suture is used, with care to ensure the superior aspect of the wrap is positioned over the esophagus or Collis segment. Only posterior aspects of the wrapped stomach should be visible if oriented and performed properly.

POSTOPERATIVE MANAGEMENT

The patient is typically extubated and transferred to the postoperative care unit or intensive care unit depending on the patient's comorbidities,

Mediastinal dissection

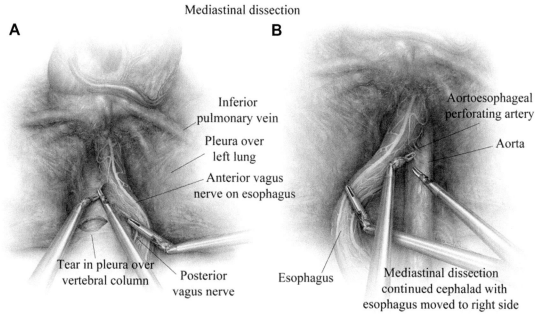

A

Inferior
pulmonary vein

Pleura over
left lung

Anterior vagus
nerve on esophagus

Tear in pleura over
vertebral column

Posterior
vagus nerve

B

Aortoesophageal
perforating artery

Aorta

Esophagus

Mediastinal dissection
continued cephalad with
esophagus moved to right side

Fig. 5. (*A*) Mediastinal dissection is continued until the inferior pulmonary vein is visualized. The left vagus nerve is readily identified and traced to the anterior vagus along the esophagus. (*B*) During anterior and posterior dissection, the mediastinal borders should always be well visualized to reduce injury to the aorta, vagus nerves, pleurae, vertebral column and the esophagus. (*From* Karush J, Sarkaria IS. Robotic-assisted giant paraesophageal hernia repair and Nissen fundoplication. Oper Tech Thorac Cardiovasc Surg. 2013;18(3):209; with permission.)

duration of the case, intraoperative complications, or urgency (elective vs emergent surgery). Most patients presenting with GPEHs are elderly with more associated comorbidities in comparison with patients presenting with gastroesophageal reflux disease in the absence of hiatal hernia. These patients are susceptible to aspiration pneumonia, myocardial ischemia, acute renal failure,

Esophageal fat pad dissection

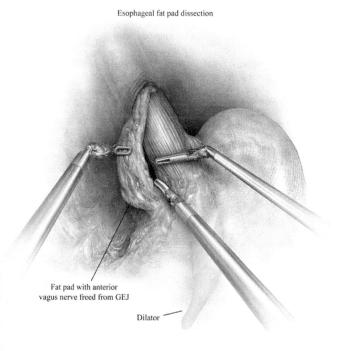

Fat pad with anterior
vagus nerve freed from GEJ

Dilator

Fig. 6. Esophageal fat pad is mobilized medially off the anterior esophagus. This maneuver facilitates visualization of the gastroesophageal junction (GEJ) and assessment of intraabdominal esophageal length. Care is taken to not injury the anterior or posterior vagus nerve. We do not routinely incorporate posterior vagus nerve in the fat pad dissection. (*From* Karush J, Sarkaria IS. Robotic-assisted giant paraesophageal hernia repair and Nissen fundoplication. Oper Tech Thorac Cardiovasc Surg. 2013;18(3):212; with permission.)

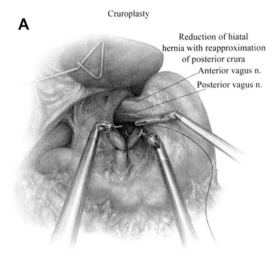

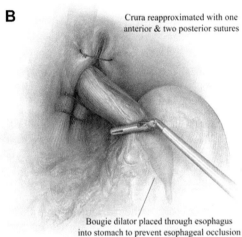

Fig. 7. (A) After adequate mobilization of both crus, a 54F bougie is inserted and visualized robotically. The right and left crus are approximated using large 0 nonabsorbable suture in simple interrupted fashion. (B) We typically place 2 to 3 sutures to close the posterior aspect and 1 to 2 sutures to close the anterior aspect of the hiatus. (From Karush J, Sarkaria IS. Robotic-assisted giant paraesophageal hernia repair and Nissen fundoplication. Oper Tech Thorac Cardiovasc Surg. 2013;18(3):211; with permission.)

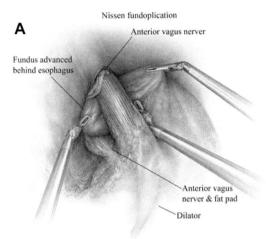

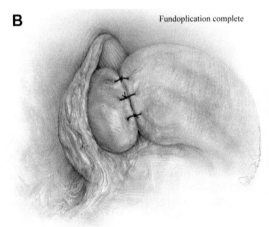

Fig. 8. (A) After mobilizing the fundus, we perform a "floppy" Nissen fundoplication with a 54F bougie in place. The gastric fundus is grasped along the short gastric dissection border using the robotic assistant arm, while the bedside assistant holds gentle caudal retraction of the body of stomach. The robotic left-hand grasper is passed carefully behind the esophagus from right to left and the fundus brought through the retroesophageal window and kept in correct orientation, with the esophageal fat pad and anterior vagus kept outside the wrap. A "shoeshine" maneuver is performed to assure a tension-free fundus. (B) 3-stitch tension-free floppy wrap of 2 to 3 cm is centered and completed over the gastroesophageal junction with bougie in place. Nonabsorbable, 2-0 sutures are placed. The proximal and distal sutures fix the fundus to the esophagus and stomach, respectively. (From Karush J, Sarkaria IS. Robotic-assisted giant paraesophageal hernia repair and Nissen fundoplication. Oper Tech Thorac Cardiovasc Surg. 2013;18(3):213; with permission.)

postoperative leaks, atrial fibrillation, and pulmonary embolism.[2] As in the literature describing the perioperative morbidity after laparoscopic approaches, the threshold to determine the presence or absence of rare postoperative leaks or hemorrhage from the Collis staple line must remain low in patients who undergo gastroplasty.

Patients ambulate and undergo a swallow esophagram on postoperative day 1. If the study is negative for a leak and postoperative anatomy is unremarkable, the nasogastric tube is removed and the patient's diet is advanced to clear liquid diet (1–2 oz/h). If the patient is tolerating clear liquids without difficulty, we advance to full liquid diet, and a soft diet over 10 to 14 days as an outpatient. All patients are reevaluated 2 weeks after surgery and then yearly with an esophagram.

Common complaints include nausea and pain. Patients are managed with an intravenous antiemetic for nausea. Pain is commonly managed with acetaminophen and low-dose narcotics in intravenous form until the barium swallow is completed, after which they are graduated to liquid forms of pain medication and discharged on nonnarcotic analgesia. Patients may remain on proton pump inhibitor or H2-blocker therapy in the early postoperative period.

Patients are discharged 1 to 2 days postoperatively and evaluated 2 weeks after discharge.

SUMMARY

Currently, no prospective studies or long-term outcome data have been published comparing the robotic approach to laparoscopic approach for GPEHs. Studies on the robotic approach for giant paraesophageal repair are limited to mostly institution specific, retrospective studies. Ruurda and colleagues[9] described their comprehensive robotic experience over a 4-year period, including type III or IV paraesophageal hernia repairs (n = 32). The median operating time was 130 minutes, the median blood loss was 50 mL, and 3 cases were converted to open technique (indication was not specified). The median hospital stay was 5 days. Draaisma and colleagues[10] described 40 patients undergoing robotic-assisted GPEH repair, with the median operating time and blood loss reported at 127 minutes and 50 mL, respectively. The median hospital stay was 4.5 days, but 12.5% patients showed anatomic abnormalities upon follow-up esophagram.

Despite the scarcity of data, we believe the advantages of robotic yield optimal visualization and significant degree of control by the operating surgeon. We notice that the operating surgeon's ability to self-first assist allows for efficient and coordinated exposure, particularly in the mediastinum. Additionally, the operator-controlled optics and robotic assistant arm allows for one assistant in comparison to the 2 additional bedside assistants commonly present with the laparoscopic approach.

Longer operative times, higher cost and technical expenses, and lack of tactile feedback are potential limitations of the robotic approach. Operative times and costs are likely to decrease with improved learning curves, and with introduction of additional industry competitors to the market. Limitations in haptic feedback do not seem to be a major factor, with adaptation to visual cues of tissue tension greatly augmenting the surgeon's perception of feel. Although prospective studies would have to be conducted to truly compare differential outcomes with these techniques, our experience thus far has been encouraging.[11,12]

SUPPLEMENTARY DATA

Supplementary data related to this article can be found online at https://doi.org/10.1016/j.thorsurg.2019.06.001.

REFERENCES

1. Fullum TM, Oyetunji TA, Ortega G, et al. Open versus laparoscopic hiatal hernia repair. JSLS 2013;17(1):23–9.
2. Luketich JD, Nason KS, Christie NA, et al. Outcomes after a decade of laparoscopic giant paraesophageal hernia repair. J Thorac Cardiovasc Surg 2010; 139:395–404.
3. Ferri LE, Feldman LS, Stanbridge D, et al. Should laparoscopic paraesophageal hernia repair be abandoned in favor of the open approach? Surg Endosc 2005;19(1):4–8.
4. Pierre AF, Luketich JD, Fernando HC, et al. Results of laparoscopic repair of giant paraesophageal hernias: 200 consecutive patients. Ann Thorac Surg 2002;74(6):1909–15.
5. Hance J, Rockall T, Darzi A. Robotics in colorectal surgery. Dig Surg 2004;21(5–6):339–43.
6. Sarkaria IS, Latif MJ, Bianco VJ, et al. Early operative outcomes and learning curve of robotic assisted giant paraesophageal hernia repair. Int J Med Robot 2017;13(1):e1730.
7. Gehrig T, Mehrabi A, Fischer L, et al. Robotic-assisted paraesophageal hernia repair-case-control study. Langenbecks Arch Surg 2013;398(5):691–6.
8. Nason KS, Luketich JD, Witteman BP, et al. The laparoscopic approach to paraesophageal hernia repair. J Gastrointest Surg 2012;16(2):417–26.
9. Ruurda JP, Draaisma WA, van Hillegersberg R, et al. Robot-assisted endoscopic surgery: a four-year single-center experience. Dig Surg 2005;22(5):313–20.
10. Draaisma WA, Gooszen HG, Consten EC, et al. Midterm results of robot-assisted laparoscopic repair of large hiatal hernia: a symptomatic and radiological prospective cohort study. Surg Technol Int 2008; 17:165–70.
11. Latif MJ, Park BJ. Robotics in general thoracic surgery procedures. J Vis Surg 2017;3:44.
12. Karush J, Sarkaria IS. Robotic-assisted giant paraesophageal hernia repair and Nissen fundoplication. Oper Tech Thorac Cardiovasc Surg 2013;18(3): 204–14.

Management of Paraesophageal Hernia in the Morbidly Obese Patient

Charles T. Bakhos, MD, MS[a],*, Shrey P. Patel, MD[b],
Roman V. Petrov, MD, PhD[a,b], Abbas El-Sayed Abbas, MD, MS[a,b]

KEYWORDS

- Hiatal hernia • Bariatric surgery • Reflux • Lower esophageal sphincter

KEY POINTS

- Morbid obesity is a risk factor for gastroesophageal reflux disease (GERD) and hiatal hernias.
- The sole repair of paraesophageal hiatal hernias (PEHs) in the obese population is associated with high recurrence rates.
- Concomitant bariatric surgery and PEH repair carries the potential advantage of improved symptom control and reduction of the risk of recurrence.
- Sleeve gastrectomy can worsen or induce GERD after hiatal hernia repair in obese patients, whereas Roux-en-Y gastric bypass can achieve better symptom control and more pronounced excess weight loss.

INTRODUCTION

Morbid obesity is a growing epidemic in the United States with a multifactorial etiology. Morbidly obese patients are defined as those with a body mass index (BMI) greater than 35 kg/m^2 with comorbidities or those with a BMI greater than 40 kg/m^2. The paradigm over the past several decades has shifted with respect to metabolic surgery in these patients. Currently, the most common surgical procedures performed for weight loss are sleeve gastrectomy (SG) and Roux-en-Y gastric bypass (RYGBP). Clinically, it is not uncommon for this patient population to present with gastroesophageal reflux disease (GERD) or dysphagia related to hiatal herniation. In fact, obesity, in particular waist circumference (a measure of central adiposity), are strongly associated with reflux disease[1,2]; furthermore, the incidence of hiatal hernias (HHs) in the obese population ranges between 20% and 52.6%.[3] These patients are challenging to manage, because the sole repair of HH, in particular paraesophageal hiatal hernias (PEHs), has been associated with high recurrence rates.[4,5] This article discusses the optimal surgical management of PEH in the obese population, with a particular focus on how to minimize the recurrence rates while controlling GERD symptoms.

PATHOPHYSIOLOGY

The surgical anatomy of PEH has been discussed in Roman V. Petrov and colleagues' article, "Surgical Anatomy of Paraesophageal Hernias," elsewhere in this issue. Although not completely understood, multiple factors are involved in the pathophysiology of obesity-related GERD and

Disclosure Statement: The authors have nothing to disclose.
[a] Department of Thoracic Medicine and Surgery, Lewis Katz School of Medicine, Temple University Hospital, 3401 North Broad Street, C501, 5th Floor, Parkinson Pavilion, Philadelphia, PA 19140, USA; [b] Department of Surgery, Lewis Katz School of Medicine, Temple University Hospital, 3401 North Broad Street, C501, 5th Floor, Parkinson Pavilion, Philadelphia, PA 19140, USA
* Corresponding author.
E-mail address: Charles.bakhos@tuhs.temple.edu

PEH. These include the chronic increase in intra-abdominal pressure, inducing the reflux of gastric contents through an ineffective lower esophageal sphincter (LES).[6] The presence of HH could further impair the antireflux mechanisms, worsening the degree of GERD.[3,7] Through a cross-sectional study using questionnaires and endoscopy, El-Serag and colleagues[8] showed that a higher BMI increases the risk of GERD and erosive esophagitis, regardless of diet and demographic variables. Similarly, Edelstein and colleagues[9] showed that central adiposity is associated with the development of Barrett esophagus. It is also suggested that obese individuals have diminished parasympathetic activity, which may affect the vagally mediated contraction and relaxation of the LES.[10] A hypotensive LES (<10 mm Hg) was the most common manometry finding (21.2%) in a series of 221 presurgical obese patients.[11] Furthermore, Pandolfino and colleagues[12] demonstrated that the altered morphology of the pressure tracings along the gastroesophageal junction promoted the formation of HHs. The intragastric pressure and the gastroesophageal junction pressure gradient, both risk factors for hiatal herniation, seem to also correlate strongly with increasing BMI.[3,8]

CLINICAL PRESENTATION

The most common GERD-evoking symptoms in obese patients include heartburn and regurgitation, in addition to dysphagia and chest pain.[13] It is, however, not unusual for patients to be asymptomatic or minimally symptomatic. Compared with 24-hour pH studies, Mora and colleagues[11] found that the presence of GERD symptoms had a positive predictive value of 69.5% in morbidly obese patients and their absence a negative predictive value of 63% only. Additionally, up to 38% of morbidly obese patients undergoing bariatric surgery were found to have an HH endoscopically.[14] Other symptoms include epigastric pain; anemia secondary to erosion of the gastric mucosa and chronic blood loss; respiratory complaints, such as aspiration pneumonia; and dyspnea. Less frequently, patients present with obstructive symptoms suggesting incarceration and/or volvulus. The physical examination may reveal decreased breath sounds or bowel sounds on the affected side of large PEHs.

DIAGNOSIS

Bariatric patients typically undergo chest radiographs before surgery that may reveal a retrocardiac air fluid level, depending on the size of PEH. Although not mandatory, a Computed Tomography

scan can help delineate the anatomy and differentiate between the different types of HH and their content. A contrast esophagogram or upper gastrointestinal series (UGI) using the right anterior oblique view is helpful in diagnosing PEHs (**Fig. 1**). Upper endoscopy with retroflexion should be performed in patients suspected or confirmed to have a hernia. The GE junction should be evaluated as well as the size of the hernia and the esophageal mucosa, looking for ulceration, ischemia, and malignancy. Endoscopic esophagitis has been found in 17% to 22% of morbidly obese patients.[8,11] Small hernias often can be missed on the preoperative work-up of bariatric patients.[1,15,16]

Manometry is useful in patients with PEH because the degree of esophageal peristalsis can in general influence the type of fundoplication performed. As discussed previously, manometry often reveals a low LES tone in morbidly obese patients, even though this may not necessarily correlate with the presence of HH.[11] Other reports in the literature showed more frequent LES relaxation intervals in this patient population.[17,18] High-resolution manometry is particularly valuable to assess the length of the HH.[13]

A 24-hour or 48-hour pH testing can be helpful in this patient population, to better quantify the degree of acid reflux. pH-metry results do not seem to correlate well with reflux symptoms or the degree of obesity.[11,19,20] As alluded to previously, central obesity rather than BMI or global obesity may explain these findings.[21–23]

SURGICAL MANAGEMENT

Unless there is a medical contraindication, the presence of PEH is in general an indication for

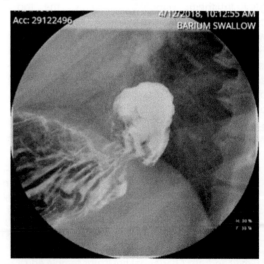

Fig. 1. Barium esophagram demonstrating a paraesophageal hernia.

surgical repair, due to the underlying potential of size increase with worsening symptoms, including GERD and dysphagia, as well as the risk of strangulation, hemorrhage, and volvulus.[24] The presence of objective GERD signs, such as esophagitis, benign stricture, or Barrett esophagus, can also weigh on the decision to intervene in minimally symptomatic patients, although most studies have not shown a protective effect of fundoplication on the incidence of esophageal cancer.[25] In obese patients, the main question is how to durably repair the hernia, whether or not to address the overweight issue, and if so how to achieve that. The different surgical options that tackle these dilemmas, therefore, are discussed.

Paraesophageal Hernia Repair Alone

The principles of PEH repair are reduction of the hernia, mobilization of the hiatus, resection of the hernia sac, intrathoracic esophageal mobilization, and reestablishing the abdominal length of the esophagus, cruroplasty, and fundoplication.[26] Morbid obesity has been shown, however, to have a negative impact on the outcomes after antireflux surgery.[5] Morgenthal and colleagues[4] found that a preoperative BMI greater than 35 kg/m^2 predicted long-term failure of laparoscopic Nissen fundoplication in a series of 312 consecutive patients. The investigators defined failure as any reoperation, lack of satisfaction, or any severe symptoms at follow-up. Although 2 other large case series showed more favorable outcomes after laparoscopic antireflux surgery in obese patients, obesity was defined as BMI greater than 30 kg/m^2 in both of these studies.[27,28] In the report by Luketina and colleagues,[28] the postoperative follow-up was standardized and included reflux questionnaire, esophageal manometry, and multichannel intraluminal impedance at 1 year but no routine contrast esophagography. Postoperative DeMeester scores, symptoms score, and LES pressures were comparable between the 2 group of patients of BMI greater than 30 kg/m^2 or less than 25 kg/m^2.

The reasons for failure are multiple and most likely due to the increase in intra-abdominal pressure with a higher gastroesophageal pressure gradient, a large hiatus, increased stress on the crural closure, and delayed gastric emptying.[4] The addition of a bioprosthesis in the repair of PEH did not seem to significantly reduce the long-term risk of recurrence in a prospective randomized trial by Oelschlager and colleagues.[29] In that study, the average BMI was 31.3 kg/m^2 in the primary diaphragmatic repair group and 30.2 kg/m^2 in the bioprosthesis group. For these reasons, a recommendation can be made that obese patients with PEH either lose weight before surgical repair or consider concomitant weight-loss surgery.

Paraesophageal Hernia Repair with Weight Loss Surgery

PEH repair with a concomitant bariatric procedure has the advantage of achieving significant weight loss, which may subsequently reduce reflux symptoms and decrease the long-term risk of hernia recurrence. Although there have been some reports of successful laparoscopic adjustable gastric banding during PEH repair, the procedure is not widely accepted in this setting due to underlying risk of band slippage and dysphagia.[30,31] Adjustable gastric banding has been increasingly abandoned as a bariatric procedure worldwide.[32] The options of SG and RYGBP procedures concomitant with PEH repair, therefore, are discussed. During their evaluation, obese patients with PEH should be counseled thoroughly regarding the impact and possible drawbacks of weight loss surgery in general. Patients may be apprehensive of the additional preoperative work-up and the expected lifestyle modifications as well as the potential for drastic weight loss and higher morbidity that may ensue from bariatric surgery.

Paraesophageal hernia repair with sleeve gastrectomy

SG was first described by Hess and Hess[33] as part of the biliopancreatic diversion duodenal switch procedure. Since then, it gained rapid popularity as a stand-alone bariatric procedure due to its relative technical simplicity and low complication profile compared with RYGBP.[32] SG causes weight loss by inducing satiety through the restrictive effect of a partial resection of the stomach and the ghrelin-producing cells.[34] Concerns were raised, however, that SG may promote gastroesophageal reflux through different mechanisms. These include the impaired signaling of ghrelin, the appetite-stimulating hormone known to increase gastrointestinal motility, as demonstrated in a rat model.[35] More importantly, the anatomic disruption of the LES by division of the sling fibers can cause further decrease in its pressure. Petersen and colleagues[36] reported this finding in 85% of patients who underwent SG, and Braghetto and colleagues[37,38] demonstrated significant reduction in mean LES resting pressure after SG, from 14.2 mm Hg $\pm$ 5.8 mm Hg to 10.5 mm Hg $\pm$ 6.06 mm Hg ($P = .01$); the length of the high-pressure zone also was affected, with 45% of patients exhibiting shortened total length

(<3.5 cm) and 70% shortened abdominal length (<1 cm). The same group followed patients 5 years after SG, and those with reflux symptoms were found to have a lower LES resting pressure compared with those without reflux. Symptomatic patients were also found to have severe acid reflux on 24-hour pH monitoring (DeMeester score 25–52), and most of them were converted to laparoscopic RYGBP.[39] Similar findings regarding the LES pressure and the DeMeester score were recently reported by Gorodner and colleagues[40] in a series of patients who underwent manometry and pH studies before and 1 year after surgery. Moreover, despite an observed 74% excess weight loss, the incidence of de novo pathologic GERD was as high as 36%. Burgerhart and colleagues[41] also reported on 20 patients who underwent laparoscopic SG with preoperative and 3 months' postoperative 24-hour pH/impedance-metry and high-resolution manometry. Although they found no increase in GERD symptoms on a validated questionnaire, esophageal acid exposure significantly increased, and the distal contractile integral as well as the LES pressure significantly decreased. They hypothesize that the new-onset GERD is caused by the disruption of the angle of His and the development of a new HH with subsequent migration of the proximal sleeve above the hiatus, as shown in **Fig. 2**. Other suggested mechanisms for worsening reflux after SG include impaired esophageal peristalsis, as demonstrated in a series of 25 patients at a median follow-up of 13 months after surgery.[42] These patients also were found to have incomplete bolus transit and an increase in the number of nonacid reflux events in postprandial periods. Additionally, the propensity for increased GERD after SG can be explained by reduced gastric compliance. This was demonstrated by Yehoshua and

colleagues,[43] who found that although the basal intragastric pressure did not change after SG, it significantly increased after the stomach was occluded and filled with saline, reflecting a substantial decrease in distensibility. This mechanism may subsequently cause an increase in gastroesophageal pressure gradient after meals, promoting the regurgitation of gastric contents. The initial increase in GERD symptoms observed at 1 year after SG seems to subside at 3 years, as reported by Himpens and colleagues.[44] The investigators speculate that as the gastric tube becomes wider and the compliance improves, the intragastric pressure gradient decreases and so does the gastroesophageal reflux. They also propose that stapling away from the left crus may cause the formation of a neofundus and a conical shape sleeve, leading to weight regain and postoperative GERD.

A recent meta-analysis reviewed 24 studies that reported postoperative reflux after laparoscopic SG: the pooled incidence of new-onset GERD symptoms was 20%, and the new-onset esophagitis ranged from 6.3% to 63.3%. Despite the heterogeneity of the included studies and the variation in the follow-up, the investigators concluded that SG can induce serious GERD symptoms among patients without preoperative reflux complaints.[45] This heterogeneity involved, among others, the size of the bougie, which ranged from 26.4F to 50F, reflecting the lack of standardization of laparoscopic SG. It could be theorized that the bougie size can influence postoperative GERD on both sides of the spectrum. On the one hand, a smaller bougie can further disrupt the angle of His and the LES pressure and cause a higher intragastric pressure; on the other hand, a bigger size bougie can limit the weight loss and increase the number of residual parietal cells.

Despite these findings, there are a few case series describing combined laparoscopic PEH repair and SG with variable success. Pham and colleagues[16] demonstrated the safety of PEH repair and SG in 23 patients, 4 of whom were known to have a hernia preoperatively. The mean follow-up was only 6 months, and the study did not address any postoperative GERD outcomes. Patel and colleagues[46] also reported 18 morbidly obese patients who underwent combined PEH repairs with SG over a 5-year period. Based on yearly postoperative UGIs and an average follow-up of 20 months, 6 of 18 patients (33%) demonstrated a small (<2 cm) recurrence, and 3 of 18 (17%) patients had evidence of reflux, which was also reflected in their GERD questionnaire scores. All patients were managed conservatively. One technical caution that the investigators discuss is the effect of chronic incarceration on the wall of the

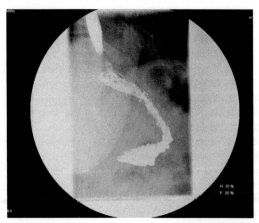

Fig. 2. UGI demonstrating a small sliding HH after a gastric sleeve.

herniated stomach that may lead the surgeon to tubularize the stomach less aggressively in order to avoid a staple line leak. On the other hand, Santonicola and colleagues[47] reported a larger case series of laparoscopic SG with concomitant HH repair (n = 78) and found persistence of GERD symptoms after surgery: 30.8% of patients had reflux postoperatively compared with 38.4% preoperatively. A recent systematic review by Mahawar and colleagues[48] included 17 studies where obese patients underwent repair of an HH (all types) along with SG. The study concluded that combined surgery is safe, but longer follow-up and direct comparison of different surgical approaches in prospective trials were necessary. Finally, a recent international survey found that only 23.3% of expert bariatric surgeons considered GERD as a contraindication to SG.[49]

Paraesophageal hernia repair with Roux-en-Y gastric bypass

An RYGBP offers multiple potential advantages that can ensure reflux control in morbidly obese patients. It induces the greatest excess weight loss among the commonly performed bariatric procedure, including SG,[50] which can subsequently cause a more significant reduction in intra-abdominal pressure. Furthermore, the small gastric pouch has minimal acid content because the acid-producing mucosa of the fundus is excluded, and the Roux limb prevents biliary reflux into the pouch and the esophagus. The loop also pulls downward on the gastric pouch, possibly reducing the risk of recurrent hiatal herniation. Finally, the classic description of gastric bypass does not alter the LES anatomy. For these reasons, RYBGP can achieve primary reflux control in morbidly obese patients. For instance, the drastic impact of this surgery on reflux esophagitis was demonstrated in a series of 100 morbidly obese patients as early as 1991 by Jones and colleagues.[51] Symptomatic GERD improvement after laparoscopic RYGBP was also found by Frezza and colleagues,[52] who reported 152 patients with documented preoperative reflux. After surgery, there was a significant decrease in GERD-related symptoms, including heartburn (from 87% to 22%), brash (from 18% to 7%), laryngitis (from 17% to 7%), and aspiration (from 14% to 2%). The use of medications also decreased significantly both for proton pump inhibitors (from 44% to 9%) and H_2-blockers (from 60% to 10%). Additionally, RYGBP was compared with vertical banded gastroplasty and was found to offer superior subjective and objective GERD control on 24-hour esophageal pH monitoring, while achieving greater excess weight loss (70% vs 46%).[53] These favorable outcomes were recently confirmed by Madalosso and colleagues,[54] who reported significant reduction of GERD symptoms in 53 morbidly obese patients after RYGBP. More objectively, patients exhibited improvement in their reflux esophagitis and a decrease in esophageal acid exposure, with the DeMeester score falling from 28.6 preoperatively to 1.2 at a median of 39 months ±7 months postoperatively.

The combined laparoscopic repair of PEH and RYGBP in morbidly obese patients was found to be safe and feasible and to achieve excellent weight loss and symptom control in a series of 14 patients (average BMI of 46 kg/m^2) by Chaudhry and colleagues.[55] The investigators reported a 68% excess body weight loss at a median follow-up of 3 years, with 33% of patients still requiring antisecretory medications for reflux control compared with 89% preoperatively. Furthermore, 78% of patients reported good to excellent quality-of-life outcomes assessed by the GERD Health-Related Quality of Life questionnaire, and an overall 89% were satisfied with their operation. The investigators did not use any mesh products to buttress the crural repair and they did not routinely perform postoperative imaging studies to detect occult recurrences. Kasotakis and colleagues[56] reported 3 obese patients with massive type III HHs and a mean BMI of 46 kg/m^2 who underwent RYGBP and PEH repair; none of the patients had evidence of recurrence on contrast studies at 12 months.

The literature also supports conversion of failed antireflux surgeries to RYGBP, particularly in the overweight or obese population. Kim and colleagues[57] reported on 45 patients with a mean BMI of 33 kg/m^2 who had failed 64 prior antireflux procedures (range 1–3 fundoplications). The anatomic reasons for failure were mainly a recurrent HH (83%) and a slipped Nissen (35%). These patients underwent wrap takedown and RYGBP, and, at 11 months' follow-up, 93.3% of them were symptom-free. This study, however, did not report objective postoperative reflux monitoring.

Despite these favorable GERD control outcomes, RYGBP carries a substantially higher rate of complications compared with PEH repair alone. These include, among others, anastomotic leakage, marginal ulcer, intestinal obstruction, internal herniation, and metabolic derangements, not to discount the long-term risk of weight regain.[58–60] Besides, a recent review of the American College of Surgeons National Surgical Quality Improvement Program database found that concomitant RYGBP and PEH repair was associated with higher morbidity, readmission rates, and reoperations in comparison to SG and PEH repair.[61]

Other reported complications in the setting of simultaneous laparoscopic PEH repair and RYGBP include pouch and Roux limb herniation into the thoracic cavity.[62] Additionally, reflux control may not be perfect after RYGBP. In a series of 47 patients with persistent GERD symptoms after RYGBP, 27 (62%) were found to have increased esophageal acid exposure (>4% with a pH <4) and 30 others (68%) an increased number of reflux episodes. The reasons for persistent reflux seem related to a substantial incidence of HHs (53%), manometric evidence of hypotensive LES (58%), and severe esophageal motility disorders (38%) postoperatively. The investigators emphasized the importance of crural closure/repair during RYGBP in patients with concomitant HHs.[63]

SUMMARY

Morbidly obese patients have a higher risk for HHs and reflux disease. The presence of PEH in morbidly obese patients represents a challenging problem. Lifestyle modification and dietary restriction should be highly encouraged in this patient population to achieve weight loss and symptom control. The pathophysiology of HH and GERD is more complex in these patients, requiring careful surgical planning to achieve a safe and durable outcome. Traditional hernia repair with fundoplication is associated with higher failure rates compared with nonobese patients. The combination of a weight-loss operation to PEH repair is emerging as a promising alternative to traditional PEH repair. Despite this, the beneficial effect of the addition of a bariatric procedure to HH repair in the obese is not clearly established. Patients should be properly counseled regarding weight loss surgery, which potentially carries a higher morbidity rate. Among the commonly performed bariatric procedures, RYGBP seems superior to SG and adjustable gastric banding, by achieving the greatest excess weight loss and the most significant reflux control.[64] SG is not advisable in obese patients with PEH, in particular those with preexisting GERD, because it can physiologically promote reflux disease. Additionally, SG may predispose to reherniation of the narrow gastric tube through the repaired hiatus. Randomized trials with postoperative objective measurements and imaging studies are necessary to better quantify the effect of weight reduction procedures on GERD and hernia recurrence in this patient population.

ACKNOWLEDGMENTS

We thank Dr. Rohit Soans for providing the **Fig. 2**.

REFERENCES

1. Daes J, Jimenez ME, Said N, et al. Laparoscopic sleeve gastrectomy: symptoms of gastroesophageal reflux can be reduced by changes in surgical technique. Obes Surg 2012;22(12):1874–9.
2. Corley DA, Kubo A. Body mass index and gastroesophageal reflux disease: a systematic review and meta-analysis. Am J Gastroenterol 2006; 101(11):2619–28.
3. Wilson LJ, MaW, Hirschowitz BI. Association of obesity with hiatal hernia and esophagitis. Am J Gastroenterol 1999;94:2840–4.
4. Morgenthal CB, Lin E, Shane MD, et al. Who will fail laparoscopic Nissen fundoplication? Preoperative prediction of long-term outcomes. Surg Endosc 2007;21(11):1978–84.
5. Perez AR, Moncure AC, Rattner DW. Obesity adversely affects the outcome of antireflux operations. Surg Endosc 2001;15(9):986–9.
6. Frezza EE, Shebani KO, Robertson J, et al. Morbid obesity causes chronic increase of intraabdominal pressure. Dig Dis Sci 2007;52:1038–41.
7. Mercer CD, Wren SF, DaCosta LR, et al. Lower esophageal sphincter pressure and gastroesophageal pressure gradients in excessively obese patients. J Med 1987;18:135–46.
8. El-Serag HB, Graham DY, Satia JA, et al. Obesity is an independent risk factor for GERD symptoms and erosive esophagitis. Am J Gastroenterol 2005;100: 1243–50.
9. Edelstein ZR, Farrow DC, Bronner MP, et al. Central adiposity and risk of Barrett's esophagus. Gastroenterology 2007;133:403–11.
10. Devendran N, Chauhan N, Armstrong D, et al. GERD and obesity: is the autonomic nervous system the missing link? Crit Rev Biomed Eng 2014;42(1):17–24.
11. Mora F, Cassinello N, Mora M, et al. Esophageal abnormalities in morbidly obese adult patients. Surg Obes Relat Dis 2016;12(3):622–8.
12. Pandolfino JE, El-Serag HB, Zhang Q, et al. Obesity: a challenge to esophagogastric junction integrity. Gastroenterology 2006;130:639–49.
13. Gyawali CP, Kahrilas PJ, Savarino E, et al. Modern diagnosis of GERD: the Lyon Consensus. Gut 2018;67(7):1351–62.
14. Dutta SK, Arora M, Kireet A, et al. Upper gastrointestinal symptoms and associated disorders in morbidly obese patients: a prospective study. Dig Dis Sci 2009;54(6):1243–6.
15. Soricelli E, Casella G, Rizzello M, et al. Initial experience with laparoscopic crural closure in the management of hiatal hernia in obese patients undergoing sleeve gastrectomy. Obes Surg 2010;20(8):1149–53.
16. Pham DV, Protyniak B, Binenbaum SJ, et al. Simultaneous laparoscopic paraesophageal hernia repair and sleeve gastrectomy in the

morbidly obese. Surg Obes Relat Dis 2014;10(2):257–61.

17. Schneider JH, Kuper M, Konigsrainer A, et al. Transient lower esophageal sphincter relaxation in morbid obesity. Obes Surg 2009;19:595–600.

18. Wu JC, Mui LM, Cheung CM, et al. Obesity is associated with increased transient lower esophageal sphincter relaxation. Gastroenterology 2007;132:883–9.

19. Suter M, Dorta G, Giusti V, et al. Gastro-esophageal reflux and esophageal motility disorders in morbidly obese patients. Obes Surg 2004;14(7):959–66.

20. Ortiz V, Ponce M, Fernández A, et al. Value of heartburn for diagnosing gastroesophageal reflux disease in severely obese patients. Obesity (Silver Spring) 2006;14(4):696–700.

21. Corley DA, Kubo A, Zhao W. Abdominal obesity, ethnicity and gastro-oesophageal reflux symptoms. Gut 2007;56(6):756–62.

22. Lee HL, Eun CS, Lee OY, et al. Association between erosive esophagitis and visceral fat accumulation quantified by abdominal CT scan. J Clin Gastroenterol 2009;43(3):240–3.

23. Nam SY, Choi IJ, Ryu KH, et al. Abdominal visceral adipose tissue volume is associated with increased risk of erosive esophagitis in men and women. Gastroenterology 2010;139(6):1902–11.

24. Ozdemir IA, Burke WA, Ikins PM. Paraesophageal hernia. A life-threatening disease. Ann Thorac Surg 1973;16(6):547–54.

25. Abbas AE, Deschamps C, Cassivi SD, et al. Barrett's esophagus: the role of laparoscopic fundoplication. Ann Thorac Surg 2004;77(2):393–6.

26. DeMeester SR. Laparoscopic paraesophageal hernia repair: critical steps and adjunct techniques to minimize recurrence. Surg Laparosc Endosc Percutan Tech 2013;23(5):429–35.

27. Winslow ER, Frisella MM, Soper NJ, et al. Obesity does not adversely affect the outcome of laparoscopic antireflux surgery (LARS). Surg Endosc 2003;17(12):2003–11.

28. Luketina RR, Koch OO, Köhler G, et al. Obesity does not affect the outcome of laparoscopic antireflux surgery. Surg Endosc 2015;29(6):1327–33.

29. Oelschlager BK, Pellegrini CA, Hunter JG, et al. Biologic prosthesis to prevent recurrence after laparoscopic paraesophageal hernia repair: long-term follow-up from a multicenter, prospective, randomized trial. J Am Coll Surg 2011;213(4):461–8.

30. Landon S. Simultaneous paraesophageal hernia repair and gastric banding. Obes Surg 2005;15:435–8.

31. Greenstein RJ, Nissan A, Jaffin B. Esophageal anatomy and function in laparoscopic gastric restrictive bariatric surgery: implications for patient selection. Obes Surg 1998;8:199–206.

32. Angrisani L, Santonicola A, Iovino P, et al. Bariatric Surgery Worldwide 2013. Obes Surg 2015;25(10):1822–32.

33. Hess DS, Hess DW. Biliopancreatic diversion with a duodenal switch. Obes Surg 1998;8:267–82.

34. Abu-Jaish W, Rosenthal RJ. Sleeve gastrectomy: a new surgical approach for morbid obesity. Expert Rev Gastroenterol Hepatol 2010;4:101–19.

35. Nahata M, Muto S, Oridate N, et al. Impaired ghrelin signaling is associated with gastrointestinal dysmotility in rats with gastroesophageal reflux disease. Am J Physiol Gastrointest Liver Physiol 2012;303(1):G42–53.

36. Peteresen WV, Meile T, Kuper MA, et al. Functional importance of laparoscopic sleeve gastrectomy for the lower esophageal sphincter in patients with morbid obesity. Obes Surg 2012;22(3):360–6.

37. Braghetto I, Csendes A, Korn O, et al. Gastroesophageal reflux disease after sleeve gastrectomy. Surg Laparosc Endosc Percutan Tech 2010;20(3):148–53.

38. Braghetto I, Lanzarini E, Korn O, et al. Manometric changes of the lower esophageal sphincter after sleeve gastrectomy in obese patients. Obes Surg 2010;20(3):357–62.

39. Braghetto I, Csendes A, Lanzarini E, et al. Is laparoscopic sleeve gastrectomy an acceptable primary bariatric procedure in obese patients? Early and 5-year postoperative results. Surg Laparosc Endosc Percutan Tech 2012;22(6):479–86.

40. Gorodner V, Buxhoever R, Clemente G, et al. Does laparoscopic sleeve gastrectomy have any influence on gastroesophageal reflux disease? Preliminary results. Surg Endosc 2015;29(7):1760–8.

41. Burgerhart JS, Schotborgh CA, Schoon EJ, et al. Effect of sleeve gastrectomy on gastroesophageal reflux. Obes Surg 2014;24:1436–41.

42. Del Genio G, Tolone S, Limongelli P, et al. Sleeve gastrectomy and development of "de novo" gastroesophageal reflux. Obes Surg 2014;24:71–7.

43. Yehoshua RT, Eidelman LA, Stein M, et al. Laparoscopic sleeve gastrectomy—volume and pressure assessment. Obes Surg 2008;18(9):1083–8.

44. Himpens J, Dapri G, Cadiere GB. A prospective randomized study between laparoscopic gastric banding and laparoscopic isolated sleeve gastrectomy: results after 1 and 3 years. Obes Surg 2006;16(11):1450–6.

45. Oor JE, Roks DJ, Ünlü Ç, et al. Laparoscopic sleeve gastrectomy and gastroesophageal reflux disease: a systematic review and meta-analysis. Am J Surg 2016;211(1):250–67.

46. Patel AD, Lin E, Lytle NW, et al. Combining laparoscopic giant paraesophageal hernia repair with sleeve gastrectomy in obese patients. Surg Endosc 2015;29(5):1115–22.

47. Santonicola A, Angrisani L, Cutolo P, et al. The effect of laparoscopic sleeve gastrectomy with or without

hiatal hernia repair on gastroesophageal reflux disease in obese patients. Surg Obes Relat Dis 2014; 10:250–5.

48. Mahawar KK, Carr WR, Jennings N, et al. Simultaneous sleeve gastrectomy and hiatus hernia repair: a systematic review. Obes Surg 2015; 25(1):159–66.

49. Gagner M, Hutchinson C, Rosenthal R. Fifth International Consensus Conference: current status of sleeve gastrectomy. Surg Obes Relat Dis 2016;12: 750–6.

50. Buchwald H, Avidor Y, Braunwald E, et al. Bariatric surgery: a systematic review and meta-analysis. JAMA 2004;292:1724–37.

51. Jones KB Jr, Allen TV, Manas KJ, et al. Roux-Y Gastric Bypass: an effective anti-reflux procedure. Obes Surg 1991;1(3):295–8.

52. Frezza EE, Ikramuddin S, Gourash W, et al. Symptomatic improvement in gastroesophageal reflux disease (GERD) following laparoscopic Roux-en-Y gastric bypass. Surg Endosc 2002;16(7):1027–31.

53. Ortega J, Escudero MD, Mora F, et al. Outcome of esophageal function and 24-hour esophageal pH monitoring after vertical banded gastroplasty and Roux-en-Y gastric bypass. Obes Surg 2004;14(8): 1086–94.

54. Madalosso CA, Gurski RR, Callegari-Jacques SM, et al. The impact of gastric bypass on gastroesophageal reflux disease in morbidly obese patients. Ann Surg 2016;263(1):110–6.

55. Chaudhry UI, Marr BM, Osayi SN, et al. Laparoscopic Roux-en-Y gastric bypass for treatment of symptomatic paraesophageal hernia in the morbidly obese: medium-term results. Surg Obes Relat Dis 2014;10(6):1063–7.

56. Kasotakis G, Mittal SK, Sudan R. Combined treatment of symptomatic massive paraesophageal hernia in the morbidly obese. JSLS 2011;15(2):188–92.

57. Kim M, Navarro F, Eruchalu CN, et al. Minimally invasive Roux-en-Y gastric bypass for fundoplication failure offers excellent gastroesophageal reflux control. Am Surg 2014;80(7):696–703.

58. Sverdén E, Mattsson F, Sondén A, et al. Risk factors for marginal ulcer after gastric bypass surgery for obesity: a population-based cohort study. Ann Surg 2016;263(4):733–7.

59. Torres-Landa S, Kannan U, Guajardo I, et al. Surgical management of obesity. Minerva Chir 2018; 73(1):41–54.

60. Velapati SR, Shah M, Kuchkuntla AR, et al. Weight regain after bariatric surgery: prevalence, etiology, and treatment. Curr Nutr Rep 2018;7(4):329–34.

61. Shada AL, Stem M, Funk LM, et al. Concurrent bariatric surgery and paraesophageal hernia repair: comparison of sleeve gastrectomy and Roux-en-Y gastric bypass. Surg Obes Relat Dis 2018;14(1): 8–13.

62. Caceres M, Eid GM, McCloskey CA. Recurrent paraesophageal hernia presenting as obstruction of Roux limb after Roux-en-Y gastric bypass. Surg Obes Relat Dis 2010;6:197–9.

63. Borbély Y, Kröll D, Nett PC, et al. Radiologic, endoscopic, and functional patterns in patients with symptomatic gastroesophageal reflux disease after Roux-en-Y gastric bypass. Surg Obes Relat Dis 2018;14(6):764–8.

64. Pallati PK, Shaligram A, Shostrom VK, et al. Improvement in gastroesophageal reflux disease symptoms after various bariatric procedures: review of the Bariatric Outcomes Longitudinal Database. Surg Obes Relat Dis 2014;10(3):502–7.

Technical Options and Approaches to Lengthen the Shortened Esophagus

Matthew G. Hartwig, MD, MHS*, Sara Najmeh, MD

KEYWORDS

• Collis • Gastroplasty • Paraesophageal • Short esophagus • Reflux

KEY POINTS

During paraesophageal hernia repair, a short esophagus is an intraoperative diagnosis that should be recognized and treated appropriately to prevent paraesophageal hernia recurrence.

- Adequate and aggressive mediastinal mobilization often precludes the need for an esophageal lengthening procedure.
- Modifications of the Collis gastroplasty are the most commonly used esophageal lengthening procedures and can be safely performed minimally invasively.
- An antireflux procedure should be performed concomitantly to a Collis to prevent symptomatic reflux.
- Total transabdominal minimally invasive approaches are the most widely used techniques today, although combined transthoracic and transabdominal techniques have been described.
- Outcomes from esophageal lengthening procedures are difficult to compare across series given the heterogeneity of the indications, techniques and measured outcomes in the literature.

INTRODUCTION

Despite the many advances made in the diagnosis and treatment of paraesophageal hernias, one of the most difficult challenges that surgeons continue to encounter is paraesophageal hernia recurrence after surgical repair, with rates as high as 60% in some recent series.[1,2] Whether these recurrences are clinically significant remains a subject of debate, but one cannot argue that a recurrence constitutes a suboptimal surgical outcome and puts the patient at risk for symptom relapse and possible redo upper gastrointestinal surgery, which carries its own risks and challenges.

Multiple factors contribute to the high rates of recurrence after paraesophageal hernia repair (PEHR). These can be divided into physiologic, patient, tissue, and technical facors.

- Physiologic factors: persistence of the pressure gradient across the diaphragm despite surgical repair of the paraesophageal hernia which continues to pull the esophagogastric junction (EGJ) and fundoplication into the chest.
- Patient factors: obesity, ascites, persistent cough, recurrent vomiting, and so on.
- Tissue factors: diminished tissue integrity or wound healing owing to advanced age, chronic steroid use, diabetes, and so on.
- Technical factors: loose crural repair, high crural tension, insufficient esophageal mobilization, or failure to identify and treat a short esophagus.

Disclosure Statement: The authors have nothing to disclose.
Division of Thoracic Surgery, Duke University Health System, DUMC 3863, Durham, NC 27710, USA
* Corresponding author.
E-mail address: Matthew.hartwig@duke.edu

Thorac Surg Clin 29 (2019) 387–394
https://doi.org/10.1016/j.thorsurg.2019.07.004

Among these contributing factors, patient- and tissue-related factors are often fixed and difficult to modify. Technical factors, however, can be optimized and should therefore be a focus of our efforts as surgeons to decrease the risk of postoperative paraesophageal hernia recurrence. Failure to identify and therefore address a short esophagus intraoperatively is one of the most cited technical factors that can lead to paraesophageal hernia recurrence after surgical repair. Failure to obtain an adequate intraabdominal esophageal length and subsequent failure to sufficiently reduce the EGJ into the abdomen to create a tension-free repair will inevitably pull the repair into the chest.

This topic has been one of the most debated issues among esophageal surgeons over the last 50 years. Some surgeons quote a high incidence of short esophagus in their practice. In contrast, others believe it to be an extremely rare phenomenon and argue that one can almost always achieve adequate intraabdominal esophageal length with aggressive esophageal mediastinal mobilization, thus making the use of esophageal lengthening procedures seldom necessary.

When looking at the literature, the quoted incidence of a short esophagus requiring an esophageal lengthening procedure is highly variable ranging from 0% to 60%, depending on the study (**Table 1**). Part of the discrepancy certainly is due

to the lack of consensus of how a short esophagus is defined.

The initial description of a short esophagus was based on preoperative radiologic studies that predict an intrathoracic position of the esophagogastric junction. Surgeons, however, quickly detected a discrepancy between the appearance of the esophagus on preoperative imaging studies and the ability to reduce the EGJ into the abdomen after maximal mobilization intraoperatively. Surgeons therefore started referring to the short esophagus as one where the EGJ cannot be adequately reduced into the abdomen intraoperatively.

The finding of such discrepancy encouraged surgeons to find better ways to predict a true short esophagus using other preoperative studies. Contrast esophagogram appearance of the esophagus as well as endoscopic and manometric measurements of esophageal length were among the most popular techniques used to try to predict a short esophagus. Unfortunately, these preoperative tools were found to be poor indicators of the intraoperative incidence of a short esophagus and their use was quickly abandoned as a predictor of the need for esophageal lengthening.[15]

Although researchers were not successful at predicting the presence of a short esophagus, some factors stood out as being associated with a higher risk of intraoperative finding of a short

Table 1
Incidence of short esophagus in the literature

Author, Year	Number of Patients	Approach	Incidence of Short Esophagus (%)
Collis,[3] 1968	420	Open	18
Gatzinsky & Bergh,[4] 1979	140	Open	37
Moghissi,[5] 1983	245	Open	39.2
Kauer et al,[6] 1995	104	Open	9.6
Csendes et al,[7] 1998	152	Open	0
Maziak, 1998[24]	94	Open	80
El-Serag, 1999[25]	1147	Open	0
Patel, 2004[26]	240	Open	96
Swanstrom et al,[8] 1996	213	MIS (lap)	14
Dallemagne et al,[9] 1998	622	MIS (lap)	0
Johnson et al,[10] 1998	220	MIS (lap)	4
Coelho et al,[11] 1999	503	MIS (lap)	0
Pierre et al,[12] 2002	203	MIS (lap)	53
Luketich et al,[13] 2010	662	MIS (lap)	63
Nason et al,[14] 2011	795	MIS (lap)	57

Abbreviation: MIS (lap), minimally invasive surgery (laparoscopic).

esophagus requiring an esophageal lengthening procedure. These factors include[16–19]:

- A prolonged history of gastroesophageal reflux disease
- The presence of Barrett's esophagus
- A history of a peptic stricture or severe esophagitis
- A history of prior antireflux surgery
- A large hiatal hernia (>5 cm) on contrast esophagogram
- Endoscopic position of the EGJ 5 or more cm above the diaphragmatic hiatus

Another fact that becomes evident when reviewing the literature is that the incidence of intraoperatively diagnosed short esophagus is not only variable across series, but also seems to be decreasing over time. This finding can be explained in a few different ways: some argue that the short esophagus was much more common in the era of open PEHR and that, as surgeons became more comfortable with laparoscopic techniques for upper gastrointestinal procedures, they also became more comfortable in performing a more aggressive mediastinal mobilization of the esophagus, which decreased the number of cases that would have been previously labeled as short esophagus owing to inappropriate mobilization. Others argue that the pathophysiology of the short esophagus stems from esophageal exposure to long periods of inflammation from gastroesophageal reflux disease, which leads to scarring and eventually transmural fibrosis, a phenomenon that used to be frequently encountered in the era of poorly controlled gastroesophageal reflux disease and peptic strictures, which are seldom seen nowadays in the era of proton pump inhibitors and improved medical management options for gastroesophageal reflux disease.

In conclusion, many questions persist around the true incidence of the acquired short esophagus in patients undergoing PEHR, but what we do know is that poor mobilization of the esophagus and inappropriate intraabdominal esophageal length during PEHR leads to a repair under tension and will significantly increase the risk of recurrence in patients undergoing surgical repair.

SURGICAL TECHNIQUE
Preoperative Planning

When planning for a PEHR, whether an esophageal lengthening procedure is anticipated should not significantly affect preoperative planning because the final decision to perform an esophageal lengthening procedure should only be taken intraoperatively after all the usual maneuvers to mobilize the esophagus have been performed. As noted, it is not typically helpful to obtain any additional workup, such as manometry or esophagogastroscopy, for predicting the need for an esophageal lengthening procedure before a planned PEHR because none of these tests are good predictors of a short esophagus and will not affect the operative approach.

Some additional preparation that has proven to be useful in our experience during a challenging anticipated PEHR include having a gastroscope in the operating room as it could assist the surgeon in confirming the position of the EGJ by transillumination at the Z line and/or the angle of His, especially in a redo surgery and in cases of a giant paraesophageal hernia. Similarly, blunt-tipped bougie dilators may serve as important tools as they may help to avoid excessive esophageal narrowing during esophageal lengthening procedures.

Preparation and Patient Positioning

PEHR are nowadays almost exclusively performed minimally invasively, with the majority of these procedures currently being performed laparoscopically and a smaller proportion being performed via a transthoracic approach. Robotic assistance is also gaining popularity for repairs of the hiatus from both above and below the diaphragm. Regardless of the specific technique, patients approached from below the diaphragm are usually positioned in the supine position and the abdomen prepped from xyphoid to the umbilicus with wide lateral exposure to allow optimal positioning of a liver retractor. The feet should be securely positioned on a foot rest to allow acute reverse Trendelenberg positioning. Some surgeons prefer the lithotomy position for laparoscopic approaches to the diaphragm. If available, a gastroscopy tower with an adult gastroscope should be on standby at the head of the bed. If gastroscopy is performed at the beginning of the procedure, one should be cautious not to use excessive insufflation because it could cause distention of the proximal small bowel and make subsequent visualization and manipulation more challenging. A transthoracic approach typically involves placing the patient in a right lateral decubitus position and entry through the left chest. This maneuver can be done via a low serratus sparing posterolateral thoracotomy or minimally invasively.

Surgical Procedure: Minimally Invasive Paraesophageal Hernia Repair with Short Esophagus

1. After establishing pneumoperitoneum, trocars are inserted in the upper abdomen and a liver retractor positioned on the left lobe of the liver to expose the diaphragmatic hiatus

2. The pars flaccida is divided to expose the right crus of the diaphragm.
3. The phreno-esophageal ligament is then divided.
4. The hernia contents are then completely reduced from the chest using a combination of blunt dissection and energy device.
5. The retroesophageal space is then created and the junction between the right and left crura is identified.
6. The hernia sac is then dissected off the mediastinum making sure to preserve the anterior and posterior vagus nerves.
7. Once the hernia is reduced into the abdomen, the gastroesphageal fat pad is dissected off the anterior wall of the stomach to clearly delineate the position of the EGJ.
8. The pneumonoperitoneum is then reduced and the position of the EGJ assessed to ensure at least 2.5 cm of esophagus is in the intraabdominal position.
   a. Pneumoperitoneum elevates the diaphragm may give overestimate the amount of intraabdominal esophageal length.
   b. If the EGJ cannot be clearly delineated, upper endoscopy can be used and the EGJ can be identified by transillumination at the Z line.
9. If the intraabdominal esophageal length is inadequate, more proximal circumferential mediastinal mobilization of the esophagus should be performed.
   a. Encircling the distal esophagus with a Penrose drain with the assistant pulling the esophagus downward toward the feet can help in the proximal mobilization.
   b. A combination of blunt dissection and careful use of an energy device ensures a safe esophageal mobilization while decreasing the incidence of mediastinal hematomas.
   c. The esophagus can be safely mobilized all the way up to the aortic arch under direct vision.
10. The pneumoperitoneum is again reduced and the intraabdominal esophageal length reassessed.
11. If less than 2.5 cm of intraabdominal esophagus is obtained after maximal proximal mediastinal esophageal mobilization, an esophageal lengthening procedure should be strongly considered.

Esophageal Lengthening Procedures

The Collis gastroplasty is the most widely accepted esophageal lengthening procedure for the short esophagus in North America. It has been performed in both open and minimally invasive settings (laparoscopically and robotically) with the goal of tubularizing the proximal aspect of the stomach along the lesser curve in continuity with the distal esophagus to create a neo intraabdominal EGJ. The initial description of the procedure by John Leigh Collis[20] was performed through a left thoracoabdominal approach and was criticized for its poor control of the ensuing gastroesophageal reflux. That original procedure has since been modified to include an antireflux procedure that usually consists of either a partial or total fundoplication. The 2 most commonly used modifications of the Collis gastroplasty are the Collis-Belsey and the Collis-Nissen.

Surgical technique: open transthoracic thoracic esophageal lengthening

The Collis-Belsey is an open transthoracic technique that was proposed and popularized by Pearson and colleagues[16,21] in the 1960s and showed excellent long-term results.

The steps of the procedure are described as the following.

1. Patient is positioned in right lateral decubitus and single lung ventilation is achieved using either a double lumen tube or a left bronchial blocker.
2. A low left posterolateral thoracotomy is performed in the sixth intercostal space.
3. The left inferior pulmonary ligament is divided and the collapsed left lung is retracted away superiorly.
4. The esophagus is then identified and dissected circumferentially then encircled with a Penrose drain.
5. The esophagus is then dissected more cranially up to the aortic arch as needed and length assessed.
6. Dissection is then carried from the diaphragmatic hiatus into the peritoneal cavity through the hernia sac.
7. The fat pad on the anterior aspect of the EGJ is then carefully dissected off and EGJ identified.
8. A 48F blunt-tipped Bougie is then advanced into the stomach by the anesthesiologist.
9. A linear stapler such as a GIA or endoGIA is then used to perform a gastroplasty the width of the Bougie along the lesser curve of the stomach.
10. A Belsey Mark IV 270° anterior partial wrap is then created using three 2.0 Silk mattress double-armed sutures placed 1.5 cm apart on the anterior wall of the stomach starting and ending on the stomach.

11. The needles on these sutures are kept intact and the sutures are left untied.
12. Interrupted 1-0 Silk sutures are then used to close the diaphragmatic crura posteriorly and are also kept untied.
13. At this point, the needles from the mattress sutures used to perform the fundoplication are carefully passed through the diaphragmatic hiatus into the diaphragm going from the abdominal to the thoracic side making sure to space them similarly on the diaphragm than on the esophagus.
14. Once all 3 sutures are passed though the diaphragm, they are tied on the thoracic side. This will reduce the repair into the abdomen and pexy it to the diaphragm.
15. The previously placed posterior crural sutures are then tied making sure not to excessively narrow the hiatus.
16. A chest tube is inserted in the left pleural space, the left lung is reinflated, and the incision is closed.

Pearson and colleagues[16] published their long-term results from 424 patients who underwent this open transthoracic Collis-Belsey Mark IV gastroplasty. The 30-day mortality in their series was 0.4%. The overall incidence of pneumonia was 4% and that of esophageal fistulas was 1.4%. In terms of functional outcomes, 85% of their patients had good functional outcomes, 9.4% had fair outcomes, and 5.6% had poor results. In this cohort, patients with peptic strictures or esophagitis with an associated motor disorder had the highest rates of poor functional outcomes.

Before the laparoscopic era, the transthoracic approach was considered central in the surgical treatment of the short esophagus because complete mediastinal mobilization of the esophagus up to the level of the aortic arch was extremely challenging through the open abdominal approach. The rise and popularization of laparoscopic surgery in the 1990s, however, created a paradigm shift in the surgical treatment of paraesophageal hernias. Enhanced visualization of the diaphragmatic hiatus and mediastinum allowed surgeons to perform safe and aggressive esophageal mobilization laparoscopically as well as confidently visualize the EGJ position and intraabdominal esophageal length once mobilization is complete. If the esophagus is deemed to be short after performing these maneuvers, lengthening procedures are then undertaken in the same setting, a procedure that was significantly simplified with the introduction of laparoscopic stapling devices, reserving the need for a transthoracic approach for the most challenging cases, such as previous failed intraabdominal repairs or long proximal strictures.[10]

Surgical Technique: Minimally Invasive Total Intraabdominal Esophageal Lengthening

Whether performed laparoscopically or robotically, esophageal lengthening procedures are usually performed concomitantly with a fundoplication. This is due to the high rates of gastroesophageal reflux noted after gastroplasty alone. A fundoplication also serves the dual role of covering the staple line of the gastroplasty and decreasing the opportunity for leak. Regardless of the type of fundoplication that is planned, however, the surgical technique of the gastroplasty is the same.

The first total intraabdominal gastroplasty technique was described by Johnson and colleagues[10] in 1998 who used an endoscopic circular stapler to create a window in the stomach through which a linear endoscopic stapler can then be introduced and the Collis gastroplasty can be performed by extending the staple line cranially toward the esophagus over a large Bougie.

A more simple way to perform the gastroplasty that is now the most commonly used technique for total intraabdominal Collis gastroplasty is the wedge gastroplasty technique. The operative steps are typically the following.

1. Once the paraesophageal hernia is fully reduced, hernia sac excised and EGJ fat pad excised, the length of intraabdominal esophagus and position of the EGJ is assessed with the pneumoperitoneum reduced.
2. If the esophagus is found to be short with inadequate intraabdominal length to allow a tension-free repair, further esophageal mediastinal mobilization should be undertaken, extending up to the aortic arch as necessary.
3. If after these maneuvers, the length of the intraabdominal esophagus is still inadequate (<2.5 cm), proceed with a wedge Collis gastroplasty.
4. A blunt-tipped bougie dilatator (typically 48F) is introduced into the stomach.
5. The assistant's right hand then retracts the gastric fundus toward the left lower quadrant and the surgeon introduces the endoscopic linear stapler through a left upper quadrant port.
6. The first staple line is directed from the edge of the fundus to the edge of the Bougie positioned along the lesser curve coming from 2 o'clock and heading toward 8 o'clock.
7. A second staple load is then introduced either through the left or right upper quadrant port to

complete the wedge gastroplasty going from the inferior edge of the previous staple line and going cranially toward the EGJ along the length of the Bougie.

8. The wedge of stomach obtained is then handed off for pathologic examination.
   a. An endo-catch bag can be used to facilitate this step.
9. A complete (Nissen) or a partial fundoplication (commonly Dor or Toupet) is then performed over the new EGJ.
10. The diaphragmatic crura are finally closed and the Bougie withdrawn.

Surgical Technique: Minimally Invasive Combined Intrathoracic and Intraabdominal Esophageal Lengthening

Combined thoracoscopic and laparoscopic esophageal lengthening approaches have also been described.[8,22] These techniques require additional transthoracic incisions that can increase postoperative pain as well as skills in video-assisted thoracoscopic surgery and therefore have not gained as much popularity given the simplicity and reproducibility of the total intraabdominal minimally invasive technique.

The combined laparoscopic and right video-assisted thoracoscopic surgery technique was described by Swanstrom and colleagues[8] in the following manner:

1. The patient is positioned in the low lithotomy position with a bump under the right scapula and the right arm extended. Double lumen endotracheal intubation is used to allow lung isolation.
2. Five ports are placed in the in the upper abdomen, pneumoperitoneum is established, and the hernia is reduced in the usual fashion as in the total laparoscopic technique.
3. If the esophagus is deemed to be short after maximal mobilization laparoscopically, the right lung is isolated and a thoracoscope is placed through a 12 mm port inserted in the third or fourth intercostal space along the anterior axillary line. A 10-mm port is then inserted in the sixth intercostal space at the posterior axillary line.
4. A blunt-tipped Bougie is inserted into the stomach by the anesthesiologist.
5. A window into the right pleura is then carefully created from the abdominal side and an endoscopic stapler is advanced from the 12-mm port into the peritoneal cavity and carefully positioned onto the lesser curve of the stomach abutting the Bougie to create a tubular stapled gastroplasty from the greater curve.
6. A complete or partial fundoplication is then created laparoscopically around the neo-esophagus.
7. A right-sided chest tube is left in the right pleural space at the end of the procedure.

Awad and colleagues[22] described a very similar operation with the thoracoscope and stapler being placed from the left chest instead of the right, which allows the creation of a stapled gastroplasty tube from the lesser curve, mirroring Pearson's technique and the minimally invasive total intraabdominal technique. There were no major complications in their patient series, the recurrence rate was 12.5%, and functional long-term outcomes were good to excellent in 87% of patients.

Immediate Postoperative Care

The postoperative care of patients undergoing minimally invasive PEHR with a concomitant gastroplasty is no different than in patients who have undergone a PEHR without gastroplasty.

There are no fixed guidelines for the postoperative management of these patients; however, our practice is to introduce clear liquids on postoperative day 1 and advance to a full liquid diet on postoperative day 2. There is no need for routine imaging for these patients and they can be followed clinically and diet advanced as appropriate.

It is not uncommon to cause a pneumothorax during extensive mediastinal mobilization, particularly in reoperative settings. When noted intraoperatively or postoperatively on chest radiographs, these are usually managed conservatively because they are usually caused by a disruption of the parietal pleura rather than a lung injury and therefore contain carbon dioxide and will reabsorb spontaneously. In rare instances where the pneumothorax is caused by a lung injury or causes significant ventilation issues, drainage via tube thoracostomy such as a pigtail catheter can be performed.

Other important aspects of the postoperative management of these patients includes controlling postoperative pain using multimodal pain regimen minimizing opioid use as well as controlling nausea because retching and vomiting can lead to tearing of the fundoplication and early hernia recurrence.

Most patients are discharged home on day 2 or 3 on a soft diet with scheduled follow-up in 2 to 3 weeks, at which time they can be advanced to a regular diet assuming there is no significant dysphagia.

Rehabilitation and Recovery

After the initial postoperative follow-up at 2 weeks, patients are typically advanced to a regular diet and can then be followed on an as-needed basis. The presence of severe esophagitis or Barrett's esophagus preoperatively should be taken into consideration and repeat surveillance endoscopy should be scheduled according to published guidelines.

For patients who complain of postoperative dysphagia at the time of follow-up, a soft diet should be continued because the dysphagia may be due to postoperative edema. These patients should be followed closely in 2 to 4 weeks to ensure that dysphagia is not related to the width of the gastroplasty or tightness of the wrap, especially if a Nissen fundoplication was performed. If dysphagia persists beyond 12 weeks, a contrast swallow should be obtained to reassess the anatomy of the repair. If the repair seems to be causing esophageal narrowing, the first step is usually EGD and esophageal dilatation. Significant dysphagia requiring takedown of the previous repair and conversion to a partial wrap is uncommon, but can be used as a last resort in patients with severe dysphagia owing to a tight Nissen.

Whether or not routine repeat imaging studies should be obtained in the asymptomatic patient on follow-up is a matter of debate. This debate stems from the observation that although radiologic recurrences on long-term follow-up after PEHR are high, these recurrences are often small and asymptomatic, and will uncommonly necessitate reoperation. These findings were highlighted in Luketich's series of 662 cases of giant PEHR where more than one-half of the patients underwent a Collis gastroplasty. These patients were followed long term (30 months median follow-up) and had excellent symptomatic improvement with significant increase in quality of life scores. In their series, 15.7% of patients had radiographic recurrence but only 3.2% required reoperation.[13] These findings were reproduced by Oelschlager and colleagues,[2] who saw an overall radiologic recurrence rate of 57% at 5 years with most recurrences being asymptomatic and only 3% of the patients requiring reoperation. The need to perform routine repeat postoperative imaging on follow-up should therefore be kept at the discretion of the surgeon with the knowledge that a significant proportion of patients may have small radiographic recurrences but the need for reoperation is actually low and should be tailored to the patient's symptoms.

Clinical Results in the Literature

An objective comparison of the outcomes and effectiveness of esophageal lengthening procedures across different series is very challenging because there is considerable variation in the indications for esophageal lengthening procedures, surgical technique, and length of follow-up, as well as the measured outcomes themselves between different studies. What seems to be unanimous across series, however, is the relatively low rates of radiologic recurrences in the long term (0%–16%) and high rates of symptomatic improvement and patient satisfaction (88%–100%)[8,10,12,13,23] in patients undergoing PEHR with a concomitant esophageal lengthening procedure. This does however come with added potential morbidity, specifically an increased risk of leak and fistulas owing to the creation of a new staple line, a risk that has been shown to be increased compared with patients undergoing PEHR without gastroplasty. Although the incidence of these leaks seems to be low in the original series ranging between 0% and 2%, the clinical implications can be devastating.[14,16,22] Moreover, the creation of a neo-esophagus from the stomach can lead to esophagitis owing to the presence of acid-secreting mucosa above the functional sphincter in continuity with the true esophageal mucosa, which can later lead to stricture.[23] Dysphagia may also occur owing to progressive dilatation of the neo-esophagus because the gastric tube lacks the normal intrinsic motility of the esophagus and will usually dilate over time, forming a nonfunctional saccular tube.

SUMMARY

Assessing the intraabdominal esophageal length and recognizing a true acquired short esophagus in the context of a PEHR is a key step in the surgical management of paraesophageal hernia and can decrease the incidence of paraesophageal hernia recurrence caused by technical factors. The rise and accessibility of laparoscopic surgery and development of endoscopic stapling devices now allows surgeons to more confidently diagnose and treat the acquired short esophagus. Aggressive mediastinal mobilization of the esophagus is often the first and only step required to address an inadequate intraabdominal esophageal length. If that maneuver is, however, insufficient to adequately reduce the EGJ into the abdomen, an esophageal lengthening procedure such as a Collis wedge gastroplasty should be performed in conjunction with an antireflux procedure. By creating a new staple line and leaving a segment of esophageal mucosa above the wrap, gastroplasties have the potential of adding morbidities to already complex procedure and should therefore be used cautiously and selectively.

REFERENCES

1. Dallemagne B, Kohnen L, Perretta S, et al. Laparoscopic repair of paraesophageal hernia. Long-term follow-up reveals good clinical outcome despite high radiological recurrence rate. Ann Surg 2011; 253(2):291–6.
2. Oelschlager BK, Petersen RP, Brunt LM, et al. Laparoscopic paraesophageal hernia repair: defining long-term clinical and anatomic outcomes. J Gastrointest Surg 2012;16(3):453–9.
3. Collis JL. Surgical control of reflux in hiatus hernia. Am J Surg 1968;115(4):465–71.
4. Gatzinsky P, Bergh NP. Hiatal hernia and shortened oesophagus. Acta Chir Scand 1979;145(3):159–66.
5. Moghissi K. Intrathoracic fundoplication for reflux stricture associated with short oesophagus. Thorax 1983;38(1):36–40.
6. Kauer WK, Peters JH, DeMeester TR, et al. A tailored approach to antireflux surgery. J Thorac Cardiovasc Surg 1995;110(1):141–6 [discussion: 146–7].
7. Csendes A, Braghetto I, Burdiles P, et al. Long-term results of classic antireflux surgery in 152 patients with Barrett's esophagus: clinical, radiologic, endoscopic, manometric, and acid reflux test analysis before and late after operation. Surgery 1998; 123(6):645–57.
8. Swanstrom LL, Marcus DR, Galloway GQ. Laparoscopic Collis gastroplasty is the treatment of choice for the shortened esophagus. Am J Surg 1996; 171(5):477–81.
9. Dallemagne B, Weerts JM, Jeahes C, et al. Results of laparoscopic Nissen fundoplication. Hepatogastroenterology 1998;45(23):1338–43.
10. Johnson AB, Oddsdottir M, Hunter JG. Laparoscopic Collis gastroplasty and Nissen fundoplication. A new technique for the management of esophageal foreshortening. Surg Endosc 1998; 12(8):1055–60.
11. Coelho JC, Wiederkehr JC, Campos AC, et al. Conversions and complications of laparoscopic treatment of gastroesophageal reflux disease. J Am Coll Surg 1999;189(4):356–61.
12. Pierre AF, Luketich JD, Fernando HC, et al. Results of laparoscopic repair of giant paraesophageal hernias: 200 consecutive patients. Ann Thorac Surg 2002;74(6):1909–15 [discussion: 1915–6].
13. Luketich JD, Nason KS, Christie NA, et al. Outcomes after a decade of laparoscopic giant paraesophageal hernia repair. J Thorac Cardiovasc Surg 2010; 139(2):395–404, 404.e391.

14. Nason KS, Luketich JD, Awais O, et al. Quality of life after collis gastroplasty for short esophagus in patients with paraesophageal hernia. Ann Thorac Surg 2011;92(5):1854–60 [discussion: 1860–1].
15. Mittal SK, Awad ZT, Tasset M, et al. The preoperative predictability of the short esophagus in patients with stricture or paraesophageal hernia. Surg Endosc 2000;14(5):464–8.
16. Pearson FG, Cooper JD, Patterson GA, et al. Gastroplasty and fundoplication for complex reflux problems. Long-term results. Ann Surg 1987;206(4): 473–81.
17. Urbach DR, Khajanchee YS, Glasgow RE, et al. Preoperative determinants of an esophageal lengthening procedure in laparoscopic antireflux surgery. Surg Endosc 2001;15(12):1408–12.
18. Gastal OL, Hagen JA, Peters JH, et al. Short esophagus: analysis of predictors and clinical implications. Arch Surg 1999;134(6):633–6 [discussion: 637–8].
19. Low DE. The short esophagus-recognition and management. J Gastrointest Surg 2001;5(5):458–61.
20. Collis JL. An operation for hiatus hernia with short esophagus. J Thorac Surg 1957;34(6):768–73 [discussion: 774–8].
21. Pearson FG, Langer B, Henderson RD. Gastroplasty and Belsey hiatus hernia repair. An operation for the management of peptic stricture with acquired short esophagus. J Thorac Cardiovasc Surg 1971;61(1): 50–63.
22. Awad ZT, Filipi CJ, Mittal SK, et al. Left side thoracoscopically assisted gastroplasty: a new technique for managing the shortened esophagus. Surg Endosc 2000;14(5):508–12.
23. Jobe BA, Horvath KD, Swanstrom LL. Postoperative function following laparoscopic Collis gastroplasty for shortened esophagus. Arch Surg 1998;133(8): 867–74.
24. Maziak DE, Todd TR, Pearson FG. Massive hiatus hernia: evaluation and surgical management. J Thorac Cardiovasc Surg 1998;115:53–60.
25. El-Serag HB, Sonnenberg A. Outcome of erosive reflux esophagitis after Nissen fundoplication. Am J Gastroenterol 1999;94:1771–6.
26. Patel HJ, Tan BB, Yee J, et al. A 25-year experience with open primary transthoracic repair of paraesophageal hiatal hernia. J Thorac Cardiovasc Surg 2004;127:843–9.

Laparoscopic Approach to Paraesophageal Hernia Repair

Ernest G. Chan, MD, MPH[a], Inderpal S. Sarkaria, MD[b],
James D. Luketich, MD[c], Ryan Levy, MD[d],*

KEYWORDS

- Laparoscopic giant paraesophageal hernia repair • Giant paraesophageal hernia
- Type 3 paraesophageal hernia • Hiatal hernia

KEY POINTS

- A successful laparoscopic giant paraesophageal hernia repair should begin with the reduction of herniated abdominal contents into the abdomen and proper entry into the areolar plane of the mediastinum.
- The second step is complete 360-degree mobilization with extensive mediastinal dissection to the level of the inferior pulmonary veins.
- The surgeon should ensure adequate tension-free intra-abdominal esophagus and properly identify the need for an esophageal lengthening procedure (Collis gastroplasty).
- Preservation of the crural peritoneal lining and integrity is key to achieving a tension-free reapproximation of the hiatal defect (with or without mesh).
- The final step is to perform an antireflux procedure or gastropexy.

INTRODUCTION

Hiatal hernias occur when there is intrathoracic herniation of abdominal contents through the hiatal orifice of the diaphragm. In normal esophageal anatomy, the gastroesophageal junction (GEJ) is typically suspended below the hiatal orifice by the phrenoesophageal ligament and posterior attachments to the GEJ and the cardia of the stomach. The phrenoesophageal ligament's elastic properties help facilitate slight movements of the GEJ cephalad, such as during peristalsis.[1] Although the exact pathophysiology of hiatal hernias remains unknown, physiologic stressors, such as obesity, chronic cough, gastroesophageal reflux, and age-related changes in tissue architecture, may cause weakening and attenuation of this ligament. This typically results in widening of the hiatal aperture, allowing for pathologic movement of the GEJ and herniation of stomach and other abdominal contents into the thoracic cavity because of increasing intra-abdominal pressures.

Hiatal hernias are generally classified into four types and are defined by the extent of herniation and its contents. The most common type is the type 1 sliding hiatal hernia (**Fig. 1**). This is defined as the simple sliding of the GEJ back and forth of the hiatal aperture. Types 2 to 4 are categorized as paraesophageal hernia (PEH), which occurs when part or all of the stomach and other abdominal

---

Disclosure Statement: The authors have nothing to disclose.
[a] Department of Cardiothoracic Surgery, University of Pittsburgh Medical Center, 200 Lothrop Street, Pittsburgh, PA 15213, USA; [b] Department of Cardiothoracic Surgery, University of Pittsburgh Medical Center and University of Pittsburgh School of Medicine, 5200 Centre Avenue, Suite 715.27, Pittsburgh, PA 15232, USA; [c] Department of Cardiothoracic Surgery, University of Pittsburgh Medical Center, 200 Lothrop Street, Suite C-816, Pittsburgh, PA 15213, USA; [d] Thoracic Surgery, Department of Cardiothoracic Surgery, UPMC Passavant, 9100 Babcock Boulevard, Pittsburgh, PA 15237, USA
* Corresponding author.
E-mail address: levyrm@upmc.edu

thoracic.theclinics.com

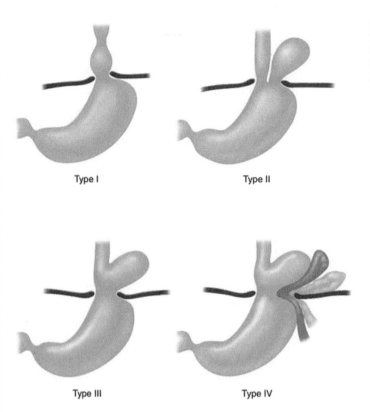

Type I

Type II

Type III

Type IV

Fig. 1. Types of hiatal hernia (types I to IV). (*From* Sun R. Esophagus. In: Imaging for surgical disease. Philadelphia: Lippincott Williams & Wilkins; 2014. p. 7; with permission.)

contents translocate through the esophageal hiatus into the posterior mediastinum. Type 2 PEH occur when the gastric fundus herniates into the mediastinum adjacent to the esophagus through an anterolateral weakness of the phrenoesophageal ligament while the GEJ remains in the normal intra-abdominal position. This type 2 PEH is rarely encountered. In the more common type 3 PEH, the GEJ and a large portion of the fundus has migrated cephalad. Type 3 PEH accounts for approximately 5% to 10% of all hiatal hernias and is associated with long-standing gastroesophageal reflux, which may lead to fibrotic changes in the esophagus causing foreshortening of the esophageal longitudinal muscles and, subsequently, the esophagus itself. This foreshortening pulls the GEJ into the posterior mediastinum, along with the proximal stomach, and may effectively lengthen the phrenoesophageal ligament and widen the crural aperture. These patients may present with obstructive symptoms including dysphagia, chest pain, postprandial bloating, or shortness of breath. Classically, a type 3 PEH with greater than 33% intrathoracic stomach has been defined as a "giant paraesophageal hernia." Type 3 PEH can develop into type 4 hernia when additional abdominal organs herniate into the mediastinum, such as omentum, colon, small bowel, spleen, and/or portions of the pancreas.

Within the last 20 years, the laparoscopic approach for PEH repair has become our preferred approach. This minimally invasive technique has been demonstrated to decrease postoperative pain, reduce morbidity, and enhance recovery when performed by experienced surgeons.[2–4] In patients with a type 3 giant PEH, operative repair is complex and challenging. Adherence to critical principles of PEH repair is essential in ensuring low recurrence rates.

SURGICAL TECHNIQUE
Preoperative Planning

Careful preoperative evaluation is critical in the successful repair of PEH. This assessment begins with a thorough history and physical examination. Currently, all patients with symptomatic PEH should be offered surgical repair. We have found that good outcomes is obtained with a laparoscopic approach even in those with severe comorbidities or advanced age. The management of asymptomatic hernia remains the subject of debate, however, and warrants further discussion. In our experience, a truly asymptomatic giant PEH is uncommon. Patient symptoms develop slowly and evolve over time, with many patients subtly modifying their lifestyles around their symptomatology. In our experience, most patients with

PEH have either typical symptoms of gastroesophageal reflux disease (heartburn, regurgitation), or obstructive symptoms including dysphagia, postprandial bloating, and chest pain. Atypical symptoms include recurrent aspiration with or without associated pneumonia, cough, shortness of breath, and dyspnea on exertion. In addition, elderly patients may deny difficulty swallowing but may present with unintentional and significant weight loss and failure to thrive because of food avoidance. Iron-deficiency anemia may also be a common in this population. Careful questioning regarding any history of blood transfusions is thus important.

Preoperative Evaluation

1. *Blood work.* This includes complete blood count to assess for anemia and serum albumin to evaluate nutritional status. There is good evidence showing that repair of large type 3 giant PEH can reverse chronic anemia.[5–8]
2. *Radiographic evaluation.* Adequate radiographic evaluation is important before operative intervention for proper planning. Typically, PEH may be an incidental finding on chest radiographs. We routinely obtain a barium esophagram for all of our elective cases (**Fig. 2**). The esophagram can provide information regarding abnormal esophageal motility and associated abnormalities, such as strictures or diverticula. Computed tomography scan is not essential, but can reveal the presence of other herniated abdominal contents.
3. *Flexible endoscopy.* We routinely perform intraoperative upper endoscopy in all patients undergoing surgical repair. This allows identification of associated pathology, such as Barrett esophagus, stricture, or esophageal diverticulae. Patients presenting emergently because of complications of giant PEH may also require endoscopic assessment to assess esophageal and gastric mucosal viability and provide mechanical decompression of an obstructed stomach.
4. *Pulmonary function testing.* Pulmonary function testing is not routinely obtained for elective repair of a large PEH. However, in patients who present with shortness of breath or dyspnea on exertion, pulmonary function tests may offer important objective information and risk assessment and rule out other pulmonary pathology. There is good evidence to suggest improvements in pulmonary function tests occur after repair of giant PEHs.[9–11]
5. *Esophageal physiology testing.* We do not typically obtain pH studies in patients with large type 3 PEHs because probe placement is

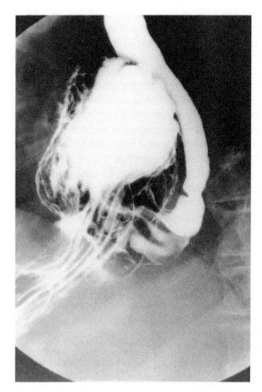

Fig. 2. Barium esophagram demonstrating a type III paraesophageal hernia. (*From* Pennathur A, Schuchert MJ, Luketich JD. Repair of paraesophageal hernia. In: Kaiser LR, Kron IL, Spray TL, editors. Mastery of cardiothoracic surgery, 3rd edition. Lippincott Williams & Wilkins; 2014. p. 342; with permission.)

difficult and inaccurate. pH testing in patients with nongiant type 3 PEHs is done selectively. Manometry is useful in the latter group of patients because it is not uncommon for this group to have ineffective esophageal motility or dysmotility. Information obtained from manometry can provide clinical information that would be used when judging the type of fundoplication to perform when choosing an antireflux barrier. Manometry in patients with giant PEH is challenging and is not done routinely in our practice.

6. *Cardiac risk assessment.* All patients undergo preoperative electrocardiogram. Patients with risk factors for coronary heart disease, including age, hypertension, history of smoking, or prior history of coronary disease also undergo cardiac evaluation with a minimum of an exercise or persantium-thallium stress test to determine whether significant coronary disease is present.

Preparation and Patient Positioning

Once informed consent is obtained, all patients undergo a modified bowel preparation with 1 L of

GoLYTELY (Braintree Laboratories Inc, A Part of Sebela Pharmaceuticals, Braintree, MA, USA). We believe it is important to avoid having patients present to the operating room with large volume of retained stool because postoperative constipation can result in postoperative bloating. In morbidly obese patients, we have found that 2 weeks of a liver reduction diet (similar to those used by bariatric surgeons) is helpful in reducing the size of the left lateral segment before surgery and thus improves operative exposure. Patients are routinely given preoperative antibiotics. Deep venous thrombosis prophylaxis is administered with 5000 units of subcutaneous heparin and sequential compression devices before induction of anesthesia. A Foley catheter is used routinely. The patient is placed in the supine position. The operating surgeon stands on the patient's right side and the first assistant on the left. The patient is positioned on the far right of the operative table to facilitate the use of a subhepatic liver retractor. A foot board is placed with adequate padding to facilitate steep reverse Trendelenburg positioning. The patient's arms are padded and angled at a 45° angle from the bed to minimize risk of stretch injury to the brachial plexus.

Surgical Approach

The laparoscopic approach to PEH repair has become the preferred approach at our institution. This procedure begins with endoscopy by the operating surgeon to assess the esophagus and the stomach. Care is taken to use minimal air insufflation during endoscopic evaluation. The stomach is decompressed and any residual gastric contents are removed. Proper laparoscopic port placement is vital to the successful and efficient execution of this operation. The surgeon needs to be cognizant of preventing displaced or dislodged ports, because the development of subcutaneous emphysema in the abdominal wall can make such cases in the morbidly obese patient difficult. We believe the key to the success and long-term durability of this repair depends on several factors including full mobilization and reduction of the hernia sac, adequate length of tension-free intra-abdominal esophagus, and preservation of crural integrity before reapproximation and closure of the hiatal opening.

In most cases, a total of five ports are used. We divide the upper abdomen from xiphoid to umbilicus into thirds (**Fig. 3**). We use an open cutdown Hasson port placement in the right paramedian line at the upper third line (usually 8–10 cm from the xiphoid in vertical distance). This port serves as the surgeon's working port. CO_2 insufflation

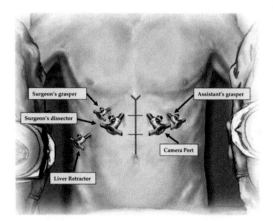

Fig. 3. Laparoscopic port placement for repair of a paraesophageal hernia. (*Courtesy of* Randal McKenzie (McKenzie Illustrations) and James D. Luketich, MD.)

and reverse Trendelenburg are then gradually introduced to allow for the patient to acclimate to these physiologic changes. CO_2 insufflation is typically raised to a maximum of 12 to 15 mm Hg, depending on the patient's hemodynamics and intraoperative stability. Once the abdomen is properly insufflated, additional ports are placed under direct visualization. The assistant's left hand typically holds the camera through a 10-mm port in the left paramedian line at approximately the same level or slightly lower to the first Hassan port. Two additional subcostal 5-mm ports are placed one hand's breath lateral to the Hassan and camera ports just below the costal margin. Lastly, a 5-mm port is placed at the far lateral right abdominal wall just below the costal margin for placement of the liver retractor. Occasionally, an additional 5-mm port is placed in the periumbilical area for additional retraction of herniated stomach as needed. As a general rule, all ports are placed roughly one hand's breadth apart to optimize exposure.

The patient is placed in steep reverse Trendelenburg so that gravity is used to maximum advantage. This assists with exposure of the esophageal hiatus.

Surgical Procedure

Step one: reduction of herniated abdominal contents into the abdomen and proper entry into the areolar plane of the mediastinum

We begin by reducing the hernia contents, such as omentum and bowel, with nontraumatic in-line graspers (**Fig. 4**). Careful attention is used with each grasp to minimize any trauma or serosal tears. The stomach is typically tethered into the mediastinum, but some of it can often be partially reduced with gentle traction to aid exposure. Use of overly aggressive grasping and traction on the

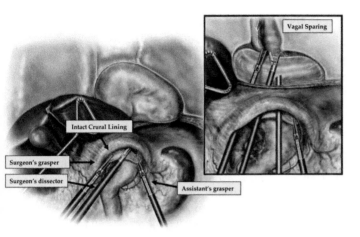

Fig. 4. Reduction of herniated abdominal contents into the abdomen and proper entry into the areolar plane of the mediastinum is performed by identifying the edge of the phrenoesophageal ligament, which has become attenuated. (*Courtesy of* Randal McKenzie (McKenzie Illustrations) and James D. Luketich, MD.)

stomach is to be avoided. Proper initial incision of the hernia sac and entry into the avascular loose areolar plane of the mediastinum is critical. We take care to avoid working within the hernia sac because this increases risk of injury to the vagal nerves. This approach also minimizes bleeding, because working from within the hernia sac can result in worse visualization from oozing of vessels in the sac. To this end, the surgeon and the assistant grasp the hernia sac just inside the hiatus at the 12-o'clock position using the surgeon's left hand and the assistant's right hand. Once the hernia sac is everted into the abdomen, the surgeon can use the hemostatic energy devices to enter the areolar plane of the mediastinum at the level of the line of peritoneal reflection.

Step two: complete 360° esophageal mobilization with extensive mediastinal dissection to re-establish normal anatomy

Once in the posterior mediastinum, a plane of areolar attachments is seen holding the hernia sac in place to the surrounding mediastinal structures (**Fig. 5**). To minimize bleeding, we recommend dividing these areolar attachments with an energy source. The hernia sac is everted off of its attachments to the pericardium anteriorly, spine and aorta posteriorly, and pleura laterally. Dissection is carried to above the level of the inferior pulmonary veins superiorly. We identify the anterior and posterior vagal nerves during these dissection maneuvers. Care is taken to avoid entry into the pleural spaces if possible. Inadvertent entry into the pleura results in CO_2 insufflation gas entry into the pleural cavity and can cause hemodynamic instability or ventilation difficulties associated with a CO_2 pneumothorax. It can also adversely impact visualization in the mediastinum because of the pleura "billowing" into the operative field. Once the sac is completely reduced

from the mediastinum, it is mobilized off of both crural pillars while taking extreme care to preserve crural peritoneal lining. Violation of crural integrity and denuding of the peritoneal lining off the crura invariably leads to exposed muscle fibers and risks injury to the crura. This can make crural reapproximation challenging and potentially increase risk of long-term hernia recurrence.

Step three: identification of adequate tension-free intra-abdominal esophageal length and assessing the need for an esophageal lengthening procedure

Once all herniated contents are reintroduced into the abdominal cavity, the next step is to identify

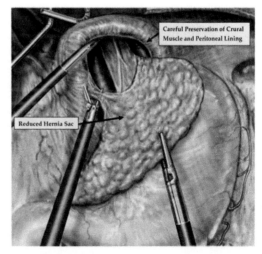

Fig. 5. Complete 360°, transhiatal mobilization with extensive mediastinal dissection to re-establish normal anatomy. Careful attention is paid to maintaining the peritoneal lining of both crus to preserve its integrity. (*Courtesy of* Randal McKenzie (McKenzie Illustrations) and James D. Luketich, MD.)

adequate intra-abdominal esophageal length (**Fig. 6**). A 2.5 to 3 cm of tension-free intra-abdominal esophagus is essential to minimize hernia recurrences. Aggressive mediastinal mobilization as previously described is critical to obtaining tension-free length. Because the attenuated and tubularized gastric cardia may look similar to the esophagus, we routinely mobilize the gastric fat pad off the stomach and distal esophagus to clearly visualize the true GEJ. We routinely perform complete fat pad mobilization so that the anterior and posterior vagal nerves are mobilized off of the esophagus. We prefer that the nerves lay outside of the fundoplication.

If a shortened esophagus is identified, a lengthening procedure is performed. We currently use a wedge-type Collis gastroplasty technique. We routinely start the Collis gastroplasty by identifying the length of neoesophagus that is needed to ensure tension-free, intra-abdominal neoesophagus. A 54F catheter bougie is inserted transorally into the stomach under direct laparoscopic visualization and is guided along the lesser curve of the stomach. A series of staple load fires are taken perpendicular down to the bougie until the bougie slides out of the stapler on closure. With gentle traction of the partially stapled gastric wedge, several additional serial firings of the endostapler are placed parallel to the bougie ("hugging the bougie") to complete the creation of the neoesophagus segment. The neofundic tip is grasped through the retroesophageal window and passed

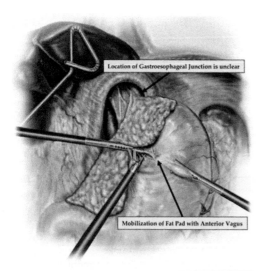

Fig. 6. The gastric fat pad is mobilized off of the esophagus and gastric cardia to identify the true gastroesophageal junction. (*Courtesy of* Randal McKenzie (McKenzie Illustrations) and James D. Luketich, MD.)

posterior to the esophagus for creation of the fundoplication, and a "shoe-shine" maneuver performed to assess appropriate orientation of the viscus (**Fig. 7**).

Step four: establish an antireflux barrier

Once the mediastinal sac is reduced, the circumferential dissection of the esophagus disrupts the integrity of the phrenoesophageal ligament and therefore the function of the lower esophageal sphincter as an antireflux barrier (**Fig. 8**). Preoperative esophageal physiologic testing and symptomatology can help guide the surgeon on the type of fundoplication to perform. Options include a circumferential "floppy" Nissen (360°), or a partial posterior fundoplication. If we are performing a fundoplication for patients with large type 3 PEH, our current preference is to perform a partial posterior fundoplication (300°–320°) to minimize side effects, such as dysphagia and gas bloat. However, the ultimate choice of antireflux barrier is determined on a case-by-case basis.

Before performing the fundoplication, several short gastric arteries are taken with the energy device. The surgeon passes a 54F catheter bougie until the largest diameter portion is seen at the GEJ. The shoe-shine maneuver is performed through the retroesophageal window, leaving the vagal nerves outside of the wrap. The assistant passes the gastric fundic tip (or neofundic tip if a Collis has been performed) to the surgeon's retroesophageal window grasper. Careful attention is paid to ensure the anterior surface of the stomach is still facing anterior and is in direct contact to the posterior surface of the esophagus (shoe-shine maneuver). The surgeon ensures the wrap is tension free. The wrap is then sutured in place with 2–0 braided permanent suture (Surgidac, Covidien) with the use of the (Endo Stitch, Covidien [Minneapolis, MN, USA]) suturing device.

In recent years, our paradigm and approach have evolved such that we do not routinely perform an antireflux procedure in all patients with giant PEH. In selected patients with exclusively obstructive symptoms, we consider a gastropexy as an alternative option. Complete, full mediastinal mobilization and complete hernia sac reduction is still required. The gastropexy is performed using a series of interrupted horizontal mattress sutures from the line of the short gastrics to an everted edge of left diaphragm. We attempt to fashion the gastropexy so as to recreate an intra-abdominal angle of His. The sutures are placed from the gastric cardia toward the fundus, sewing to a fold of the left diaphragm that lies above the spleen. The gastropexy stomach thus lies along a virtual line where the short gastric

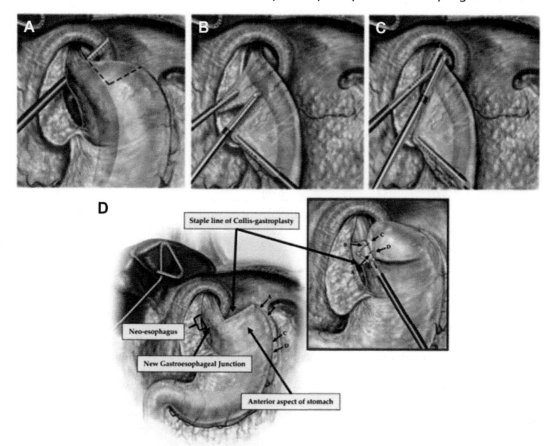

Fig. 7. In the setting of a shortened esophagus, a wedge collis gastroplasty is performed (*A–C*). In (*D*), points A–D represent the line of the transected short gastric arteries of the neofundic tip that is grasped through the retro-esophageal window and passed posterior to the esophagus for creation of the fundoplication, and a "shoe-shine" maneuver performed to assess appropriate orientation of the wrap. (*Courtesy of* Randal McKenzie (McKenzie Illustrations) and James D. Luketich, MD.)

vessels normally reside, thereby simulating a normal anatomic lie of the stomach.

Step five: closure and reapproximation of the diaphragmatic defect (with or without mesh)

Once the fundoplication is secure, next step is closure and reapproximation of the hiatal defect (see **Fig. 8**). We recommend a tension-free primary suture closure of the hiatus. Because the crura are frequently attenuated in patients with PEH, the success of this of this step is dependent on several factors including the preservation of the peritoneal lining of the crura during the hiatal dissection and the full mobilization of the crura from the surrounding structures. This includes division of the spleno-diaphragmatic attachments along the left crus as an important part of ensuring tension-free diaphragm closure. We typically place two posterior sutures with 0-Surgidac and an anterior suture or lateral suture. In patients with a very splayed hiatal opening or a giant PEH, we often induce a deliberate CO_2 pneumothorax in the left pleural space

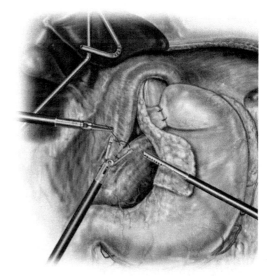

Fig. 8. Primary repair and reapproximation of the right and left crus is performed using the endostitch device. (*Courtesy of* Randal McKenzie (McKenzie Illustrations) and James D. Luketich, MD.)

Table 1
Large retrospective series that reported surgical and radiologic recurrences following laparoscopic repair of their giant paraesophageal hernia

Reference (Year)	N	Follow-up (mo)	30-d Mortality	Surgical Recurrence (%)	Radiologic Recurrence (%)
Sorial et al,[15] 2019	204	nr	0 (0)	nr	nr
Chang & Thackeray,[16] 2016	221	14.5	1 (0.5)	1 (0.5)	2/221 (3.6)
Dallemagne et al,[17] 2011	85	118	0 (0)	2 (1.7)	23/35 (65.7)
Luketich et al,[18] 2010	662	30	11/662 (1.7)	21 (3.2)	70/445 (15.7)
Zaninotto et al,[19] 2007	54	71	0 (0)	5 (9.3)	11/53 (20.8)
Aly et al,[20] 2005	100	nr	0 (0)	4 (4.0)	14/60 (23.3)
Mattar et al,[4] 2002	136	40	3 (2.2)	3 (2.2)	14/32 (43.8)
Jobe et al,[21] 2002	52	39	0 (0)	2 (3.8)	11/34 (32.4)
Hashemi et al,[22] 2000	27	24	0 (0)	nr	9/21 (42.9)

Abbreviation: nr, not reported.

to allow for tension-free diaphragm closure. This is performed by placing a 5-mm port into the left chest under direct visualization and instilling CO_2 gas. This creates a floppy diaphragm on the left and usually allows the surgeon to reapproximate the crura without tension. We use a similar technique to assist with the initial gastropexy sutures when performing a gastropexy. Alternatively, one could dramatically decrease the CO_2 abdominal insufflation pressure, but this impairs visualization of the hiatus while suturing. Once the hiatus is reapproximated, a grasper should easily be introduced through the hiatus to ensure the closure is not too tight because that can also be a source of postoperative dysphagia or pseudoachalasia. A nasogastric tube is advanced under direct visualization before the removal of abdominal insufflation and the conclusion of the case.

The use of mesh buttress of the hiatal closure is a controversial subject of many prior publications.[12–14] In our experience, the routine use of mesh is not necessary. We believe that critical attention to the tenets of preserving crural integrity, aggressive mediastinal mobilization, and ensuring tension-free intra-abdominal esophagus is more important in minimizing recurrences than the placement of mesh. Mesh prosthesis pose risks of infection, erosion, and tissue fibrosis (which can lead to dysphagia or pseudoachalasia picture). Thus, we use bioprosthetic mesh reinforcement in only selected cases where primary repair is not deemed feasible.

Immediate Postoperative Care

The patient is typically extubated in the operating room. Most patients are cared for in a step-down unit in the postoperative period. Patients are started on scheduled antiemetics and simethicone to prevent gas bloating. We typically keep the nasogastric tube in place overnight. All patients undergo a barium esophagram postoperatively to confirm intact repair, absence of leak, and free flow of contrast into the stomach. Patients are then started on a clear liquid diet and advanced accordingly. A staff nutritionist and dietician meet with patients before discharge to enhance diet compliance and education. We attempt to minimize narcotics in the postoperative period because these drugs exacerbate constipation and bloating.

REHABILITATION AND RECOVERY

On discharge, patients are instructed to a full liquid intake after 3 days and then soft solids until the postoperative clinic visit, which occurs in 2 weeks. Patients are instructed to eat smaller meals at a higher frequency (five small meals daily) to minimize the risk of gas bloat and dysphagia.

CLINICAL RESULTS IN THE LITERATURE

Table 1 provides large retrospective series that reported surgical and radiologic recurrences following laparoscopic repair of giant PEH.

SUMMARY

The repair of PEH is a complex operation that requires careful attention to several key elements to achieve a successful repair. In 1998, Pearson and colleagues[23] published results of their transthoracic approach with a thoracotomy and fundoplication with esophageal lengthening as needed for repair of PEH. This series remains the gold standard in terms of long-term outcomes and recurrence rates. In the modern era of minimally invasive surgery, the laparoscopic approach to PEH repair has become the standard. To reproduce the landmark results of Pearson and colleagues, surgeons should adhere to the following principles of repair:

- Complete mobilization of the hernia sac and reduction from the chest
- Tension-free reduction of the stomach and other herniated intra-abdominal contents to the abdomen with preservation of both vagal nerves
- Accurate, careful assessment for esophageal shortening and the appropriate use of the Collis gastroplasty as needed to create 2.5 to 3 cm of tension-free intra-abdominal esophagus (or neoesophagus)
- Preservation of the crural integrity and peritoneal lining
- Proper construction of a fundoplication tailored for each patient based on their symptomatology and manometry (when available)

REFERENCES

1. Kwok H, Marriz Y, Al-Ali S, et al. Phrenoesophageal ligament re-visited. Clin Anat 1999;12:164–70.
2. Luketich JD, Raja S, Fernando HC, et al. Laparoscopic repair of giant paraesophageal hernia: 100 consecutive cases. Ann Surg 2000;232:608–18.
3. Karmali S, McFadden S, Mitchell P, et al. Primary laparoscopic and open repair of paraesophageal hernias: a comparison of short-term outcomes. Dis Esophagus 2008;21:63–8.
4. Mattar SG, Bowers SP, Galloway KD, et al. Long-term outcome of laparoscopic repair of paraesophageal hernia. Surg Endosc 2002;16:745–9.
5. Carrott PW, Markar SR, Hong J, et al. Iron-deficiency anemia is a common presenting issue with giant paraesophageal hernia and resolves following repair. J Gastrointest Surg 2013;17:858–62.
6. Hayden JD, Jamieson GG. Effect on iron deficiency anemia of laparoscopic repair of large paraesophageal hernias. Dis Esophagus 2005;18:329–31.
7. Lebenthal A, Waterford SD, Fisichella PM. Treatment and controversies in paraesophageal hernia repair. Front Surg 2015;2:13.
8. Skipworth RJE, Staerkle RF, Leibman S, et al. Transfusion-dependent anaemia: an overlooked complication of paraoesophageal hernias. Int Sch Res Notices 2014;2014:4.
9. Carrott PW, Hong J, Kuppusamy M, et al. Repair of giant paraesophageal hernias routinely produces improvement in respiratory function. J Thorac Cardiovasc Surg 2012;143:398–404.
10. Low DE, Simchuk EJ. Effect of paraesophageal hernia repair on pulmonary function. Ann Thorac Surg 2002;74:333–7.
11. Wirsching A, Klevebro F, Boshier PR, et al. The other explanation for dyspnea: giant paraesophageal hiatal hernia repair routinely improves pulmonary function. Dis Esophagus 2019. [Epub ahead of print].
12. Oelschlager BK, Pellegrini CA, Hunter J, et al. Biologic prosthesis reduces recurrence after laparoscopic paraesophageal hernia repair: a multicenter, prospective, randomized trial. Ann Surg 2006;244:481–90.
13. Oelschlager BK, Pellegrini CA, Hunter JG, et al. Biologic prosthesis to prevent recurrence after laparoscopic paraesophageal hernia repair: long-term follow-up from a multicenter, prospective, randomized trial. J Am Coll Surg 2011;213:461–8.
14. Stavropoulos G, Flessas II, Mariolis-Sapsakos T, et al. Laparoscopic repair of giant paraesophageal hernia with synthetic mesh: 45 consecutive cases. Am Surg 2012;78:432–5.
15. Sorial RK, Ali M, Kaneva P, et al. Modern era surgical outcomes of elective and emergency giant paraesophageal hernia repair at a high-volume referral center. Surg Endosc 2019. [Epub ahead of print].
16. Chang CG, Thackeray L. Laparoscopic hiatal hernia repair in 221 patients: outcomes and experience. JSLS 2016;20 [pii:e2015.00104].
17. Dallemagne B, Kohnen L, Perretta S, et al. Laparoscopic repair of paraesophageal hernia. Long-term follow-up reveals good clinical outcome despite high radiological recurrence rate. Ann Surg 2011;253(2):291–6.
18. Luketich JD, Nason KS, Christie NA, et al. Outcomes after a decade of laparoscopic giant paraesophageal hernia repair. J Thorac Cardiovasc Surg 2010;139:395–404, 404.e391.
19. Zaninotto G, Portale G, Costantini M, et al. Objective follow-up after laparoscopic repair of large type III hiatal hernia. Assessment of safety and durability. World J Surg 2007;31:2177–83.
20. Aly A, Munt J, Jamieson GG, et al. Laparoscopic repair of large hiatal hernias. Br J Surg 2005;92:648–53.
21. Jobe BA, Aye RW, Deveney CW, et al. Laparoscopic management of giant type III hiatal hernia and short esophagus. Objective follow-up at three years. J Gastrointest Surg 2002;6:181–8 [discussion: 188].
22. Hashemi M, Peters JH, DeMeester TR, et al. Laparoscopic repair of large type III hiatal hernia: objective followup reveals high recurrence rate. J Am Coll Surg 2000;190:553–60 [discussion: 560–1].
23. Maziak DE, Todd TR, Pearson FG. Massive hiatus hernia: evaluation and surgical management. J Thorac Cardiovasc Surg 1998;115:53–60 [discussion: 61–2].

Short-Term and Long-Term Outcomes of Paraesophageal Hernia Repair

Anne-Sophie Laliberte, MD, FRCSC[a], Brian E. Louie, MD, MHA, MPH, FRCSC[b],*

KEYWORDS

- Paraesophageal hernia • Laparoscopic • Fundoplication • Short-term and long-term outcomes

KEY POINTS

- Laparoscopic paraesophageal hernia repair results in excellent overall patient satisfaction and improved quality of life.
- Radiologic recurrences can be reduced by reducing tension with use of a lengthening procedure and mesh reinforcement.
- Repair usually resolves both signs and symptoms of gastroesophageal reflux, anemia, obstruction and shortness of breath.
- There is a lack of very long-term outcomes over 10 years.

INTRODUCTION

The assessment of outcomes after surgical repair of a paraesophageal hernia (PEH) is a difficult and complex problem. One component of the complexity is the anatomic defect through which a wide variation of herniated contents can be found. Another component is the associated symptom(s) that patients experience that, to a certain extent, are dependent on the hernia's size, configuration, and type of repair. Lastly, there is a wide range of reported outcomes that are not consistently defined and are influenced heavily by the outcome definition and how it is measured.

This article focuses on the short-term ($\leq$ 5 years) and long-term (>5 years) outcomes after a PEH repair defined as an axial separation from gastroesophageal junction (GEJ) and diaphragmatic hiatus by at least 5 cm. Additionally, more than one-third of the stomach must reside in the thoracic cavity and the fundus located above the GEJ. This article focuses on outcomes from laparoscopic repairs because they are currently the predominant approach but have included some comparative analysis to open repairs.

ASSESSMENT OF OUTCOMES

The success or failure of PEH repair is difficult to define because it depends on the outcome selected and the perspective of the evaluator.[1,2] A comprehensive analysis of the outcomes requires compartmentalization to be able to completely assess the success or failure of the repair.[3] A review of the literature shows that there are no consistently used outcomes when it comes to assessing PEH repair. Moreover, the literature often includes patients with sliding hernias who have symptomatic gastroesophageal reflux disease (GERD). What is clear is that outcomes should be assessed across several domains and

Disclosure Statement: A.-S. Laliberte has no disclosures. Dr B.E. Louie discloses relationships with: Intuitive Surgical, Torax/Ethicon J and J.
[a] Division of Thoracic Surgery, Swedish Medical Center, 1101 Madison Street, Suite 900, Seattle, WA 98104, USA; [b] Division of Thoracic Surgery, Swedish Medical Center, Swedish Digestive Health Institute, 1101 Madison Street, Suite 900, Seattle, WA 98104, USA
* Corresponding author.
E-mail address: Brian.Louie@swedish.org

Thorac Surg Clin 29 (2019) 405–414
https://doi.org/10.1016/j.thorsurg.2019.07.005
1547-4127/19/© 2019 Elsevier Inc. All rights reserved.

thoracic.theclinics.com

involve both subjective and objective outcomes to provide a comprehensive understanding.

For the purposes of this review, the outcomes reviewed include both short-term (<5-year) and long-term (>5-year) data. Perioperative morbidity and mortality are excluded because they are covered in another section. The broad assessment includes

- Patient-reported outcomes
  - GERD related
    - Typical
    - Atypical
  - Non–GERD related
    - Pulmonary
    - Hematologic
    - Obstructive
- Radiologic recurrence
- Additional therapy or interventions
- Objective measurements (where applicable)
  - pH testing
  - Pulmonary function
  - Hemoglobin and hematocrit levels for anemia

PATIENT-REPORTED OUTCOMES
Gastroesophageal Reflux Disease–Related Symptoms

It is not surprising that heartburn and regurgitation are commonly associated symptoms in patients with PEHs. These symptoms are increasingly demonstrated as the size of the hernia increases. Unlike non-GERD symptoms (discussed later), which respond to simple reduction of the hernia and repair of the hiatal opening, this strategy results in only 50% resolution of the GERD symptoms.[4] To achieve complete resolution of the GERD symptoms, it is necessary to combine hernia repair with a fundoplication.

Several studies documented the specific symptoms of heartburn and regurgitation and found that these were seen in at least 50% of their study populations.[2,5,6] After repair there was significant improvement in each of these specific symptoms between 1 year and 3 years of follow-up. Similarly, Parameswaran and colleagues[7] found that pain and reflux were present in approximately 50% of PEH patients. They also used the Gastrointestinal Symptom Rating Scale to evaluate pain and reflux prerepair and postrepair and showed significant improvement in these symptoms.

The presence of atypical symptoms in patients with a PEH is focused on chest pain, and few if any studies specifically looked at globus, laryngitis, hoarseness, or chronic cough. There are several possible explanations. First, the symptoms

do exist but are much overshadowed by the other classic symptoms. Second, once the paraesophageal configuration (fundus above GEJ) appears, the reconstituted acute angle of His creates enough of an antireflux barrier to lessen the appearance of these symptoms.

Other studies have used a variety of patient-reported outcome questionnaires, such as the GERD-Health Related Quality of Life (GERD-HRQL) questionnaire (**Table 1**). These same studies along with several others also demonstrate improvements in GERD-HRQL and overall success in short-term outcomes between laparoscopic and open paraesophageal repair.[8] Overall satisfaction and the clinical symptomatic improvement are maintained between 1 year and 5 years. Proton pump inhibitors (PPIs) are resumed modestly in some series and in other series are resumed approximately 50% of the time (**Tables 2 and 3**).

The use of postoperative pH testing is much more common in patients with GERD and uncommonly used after PEH repair. It is generally accepted that patient complaints of GERD symptoms do not necessarily correlate with objective evidence of GERD on pH testing.[26] In patients undergoing Nissen fundoplication for GERD, Granderath[27] compared the DeMeester score preoperatively, at 3 months and at 1 years, and showed there was no acid exposure after the surgery. Wiechmann and colleagues,[28] however, compared pH studies preoperatively and 1-year postoperatively and showed a significant decrease of pH below 5 after laparoscopic PEH, and Levy and colleagues[25] showed normalization of the DeMeester score after a combined Nissen and Hill procedure.

Multiple studies focusing on long-term clinical outcomes assessment report clinical improvement after surgery maintained for 5 or more years.[10,11,25,29] (see **Table 3**). The overall satisfaction after PEH repair is approximately 90% and durable over time.[22,30] The improvement of quality of life after the surgery seems to persist over years. The proportion of patients reporting symptoms of GERD was decreased postoperatively and was similar between 1-year and 10-year follow-up.[24] All different types of PEH repair showed GERD-HRQL improvement after surgery that is maintained over the long term.[31]

There is a lack of very long-term follow-up after paraesophageal repair in the literature and there seems to be few satisfactory data over 10 years. Extrapolation from the GERD literature may be inferred from the 2 studies reporting more than 10-year outcomes in antireflux procedures. Aye and colleagues[32] reported a 9.1% rate of PEH

Table 1
Summary gastroesophageal reflux disease and dysphagia clinical assessment tool

Tool	Description
GERD-HRQL score[9]	Nine items with a score ranging from 0 (no symptoms) to 50 (incapacitating in all): 1. How bad is your heartburn? 2. Heartburn when lying down? 3. Heartburn when standing up? 4. Heartburn after meals? 5. Does heartburn change your diet? 6. Does heartburn change your sleep? 7. Do you have difficulty swallowing? 8. Do you have pain swallowing? 9. Do you have bloating of gassy feeling? 10. If you are taking medication, does it affect your daily life? 11. How satisfied are you with your present condition?
QOLRAD[10]	Five subscales: emotional distress (6 items), sleep disturbance (5 items), food/drink problems (6 items), physical/social functioning (5 items), and vitality (3 items). Measure GERD and overall success. The maximum score is 7, with higher score representing a better quality of life.
Gastrointestinal Quality of Life Index[11]	Thirty-six items scored on a 5-point Likert scale (range, 0–144). The higher the score is, the better the quality of life. Five subscales: gastrointestinal symptoms, emotional status, physical function, social function, and stress by medical treatment
Gastrointestinal Symptom Rating Scale (GSRS)[12]	The GSRS contains 15 items, each rated on a 7-point Likert scale from no discomfort to very severe discomfort. Five subscales: abdominal pain, reflux syndrome, diarrhea syndrome, indigestion syndrome, and constipation syndrome.
DSS[10]	Dysphagia questionnaire assessing the ability to ingest a range of common solid and liquid food items. The maximum score is 45, with the higher score representing better ability to swallow food.

recurrence after 25 years, whereas Robinson and colleagues[33] did not report the rate of recurrence after 20 years of follow-up.

Non–Gastroesophageal Reflux Disease–Related Symptoms

PEHs, as opposed to smaller, sliding hiatal hernias, often produce a variety of non–GERD-like symptoms. These are due to the mass effect of the hernia on neighboring structures, such as the lung (respiratory), to its shape and relative position to the hiatal canal (obstruction) and to motion within the hiatal canal (anemia).

Respiratory Symptoms

Respiratory-related symptoms in the presence of a PEH are predominately shortness of breath. Asthma-like symptoms, recurrent bronchitis, and pneumonia, often secondary to aspiration, are all associated as well. Intuitively, reduction of the herniated contents causing less compression on the lungs should lead to improvement in breathing status. The mechanism may be more complicated, however, and involve regional ventilation/perfusion mismatching from compression and possible direct cardiac compression.[34] Additionally, reduction of any amount of refluxate reaching the airway is also likely to result in improved lung function.

Lidor and colleagues,[16] using a validated GERD quality-of-life score subcomponent asking about shortness of breath, showed clinical improvement of the respiratory symptoms over a 3-year period. There is only 1 study that evaluated respiratory outcomes in patients with pulmonary function testing. It showed significant improvements in forced expiratory volume in 1 second (FEV_1) and forced vital capacity (FVC) in terms of percent improvement and percent-predicted values. A nonsignificant improvement was seen in diffusing capacity for carbon dioxide. Two patients who were on home oxygen were able to discontinue their home oxygen postoperatively. Most importantly, the hernia size correlated with the degree of improvement with an improvement in FEV_1 of 19.6% and FVC of 19.7% when the entire stomach was intrathoracic.[35]

Table 2
Early outcomes after paraesophageal hernia repair (6 months–5 years)

Articles	Mean Follow-up (mo)	Radiological Recurrence (%)	Redo Surgery (%)	Reintroduction of Proton Pump Inhibitor (%)	Recurrence of Symptoms (%)	Overall Satisfaction (%)
Oelschlager et al,[13] 2011	6	14	—	11–17	—	—
Luketich et al,[6] 2000	12	—	1	10	—	91
Pierre et al,[14] 2002	18	—	2.5	16	—	93
Luketich et al,[15] 2010	30	15.7[a]	3.28[a]	—	—	90
Lidor et al,[16] 2015	36	27[b]	3.6	—	—	—
Jobe et al,[17] 2002	39	32	5	14	19	—
Oelschlager et al,[13] 2011	58	54–59	3.5	44–45	—	—
Nason et al,[18] 2008	44	15	4.4	35	—	86.7
Oelschlager et al,[19] 2012	58	57	3	44	—	—

[a] 30 days.
[b] 1 year.

Table 3
Long-term outcomes after paraesophageal hernia repair (>5 years)

Articles	Mean Follow-up (mo)	Radiological Recurrence (%)	Redo Surgery (%)	Reintroduction of Proton Pump Inhibitor(%)	Recurrence of Symptoms (%)	Overall Satisfaction (%)
Gryska and Vernon,[20] 2005	62	—	0.8	8	—	86
Simorov et al,[21] 2014	70	33.9	0.9	34	16	—
Lafullarde et al,[22] 2001	72	—	7.3	11	23	90
Merzlikin et al,[10] 2017	89	13	0	26	—	—
Targorona et al,[23] 2013	107	46	—	13	21	—
Dallemagne et al,[11] 2011	118	66	3	—	—	—
White et al,[24] 2008	135	32	6.45	—	—	—
Levy et al,[25] 2017 Hybrid group	61	5	2.6	5	—	—
Levy et al,[25] 2017 Nissen group	62	42	9.7	23	—	—

Only 1 study reported long-term significant improvement and durability in respiratory symptoms, including cough, asthma, and dyspnea, at a median follow-up of 118 months.[11]

Hematologic Symptoms

The association of anemia and PEHs was first reported in 1931.[36] Since then, 5 studies have been completed examining the effect of repair on anemia (**Table 4**). A vast majority of patients usually present with fatigue, shortness of breath, and lack of stamina and are found to be anemic. Rarely have patients presented with frank bleeding. The hematologic symptoms included chronic and acute anemia or active bleeding. A variety of outcomes measures have been tracked in this situation, including resolution of anemia, improvement in hemoglobin or hematocrit, and discontinuation of supplemental iron therapy.

Resolution of anemia after repair of the PEH is achieved in 60% to 100% of patients. Carrott and colleagues[42] in the largest published series to date reported that 71% of patients had resolution of anemia after hiatal hernia repair. Comparatively, the smallest series of 11 had 100% resolution of the anemia.[39] All studies reporting improvement in hemoglobin levels showed a significant improvement and similarly there was a high rate of iron therapy discontinuation. Unfortunately, the "normal" hemoglobin definition varied in these older studies. In addition, the studies did not all account for the use of preoperative anemia therapy.

The most commonly accepted etiology for the anemia is caused by the venous congestion at the neck of the hernia causing chronic bleeding.[41] This often is associated with the presence of a Cameron's ulcer, which is present in varying ranges in published series. Resolution of the anemia seems likely when Cameron's ulcer are identified preoperatively than when absent. But the absence of a Cameron ulcer should not be used as an argument that a patient's anemia is not related to the presence of a PEH.

Resolution of anemia seems durable in the 1 long-term outcome study.[11]

Obstructive Symptoms

One of the more common presentations of a PEH is postprandial chest pain/discomfort, which signals some form of obstruction as the cause of the symptoms. Often this is also associated with early satiety as patients try to adjust to the presence of the herniated and partially obstructed stomach. These 2 symptoms usually are due to obstruction of the herniated stomach secondary to volvulus and improve in almost all cases with reduction of the hernia.[2,5,6] Patients also can present with preoperative dysphagia, which can be attributed to the hiatal hernia, particularly if the hernia cause distortion of the GEJ.[11] The symptoms also are significantly improved after repair.[2,6]

ADDITIONAL OUTCOMES
Radiologic Recurrence

One of the more controversial outcomes after PEH repair remains the identification of a radiologic recurrence. During transition from open to laparoscopic repair, recurrence was defined as any identified herniation on a videofluoroscopy study. Using this definition, Hashemi and colleagues[43] reported a recurrence rate of 42% after laparoscopic repair compared with 15% in the open group. The definition of radiologic recurrence has changed over time and now it is common to see a definition where any vertical recurrence of greater than 2 cm

Table 4
Anemia and paraesophageal hernia

Authors	n	Cameron Ulcers (%)	Transfusion	Resolution of Anemia (%)	Improvement (%)
Carrott et al,[37] 2013	77	32	—	71	90% rise postoperative hemoglobin 73% discontinuation iron therapy
Haurani et al,[38] 2012	62	26	—	60	70% improvement postoperative hemoglobin
Hayden and Jamieson,[39] 2005	11	—	—	100	1 patient resumed his iron therapy
Trastek et al,[40] 1996	49	—	65% 6 units (2–70)	91.8	—
Windsor and Collis,[41] 1967	59	8.5%	—	—	Increase in hemoglobin 5.4 g/100 mL No recurrence

is a recurrence because it is associated with higher symptomatic change.[2,13,15,44]

Radiologic recurrence or anatomic recurrence rates range from 7% to 66% across a wide variety of studies that include varying rates of mesh and Collis gastroplasty (**Table 5**). In 1 of the largest series, Luketich and colleagues[15] reported a radiologic (<2 cm) recurrence rate of 16% after hiatal hernia repair with primary closure of the hiatus, a low rate of crural mesh (13%) but the highest rate of esophageal lengthening procedures (63%). Similarly, Zehetner and colleagues[45] reported a 12% recurrence (any) rate with a higher rate of crural mesh (84%) and a modest rate of esophageal lengthening (40%). In studies where axial tension addressed at much lower rates, the radiologic recurrence rates are higher.[11,13,23] These studies highlight 2 key principles in the management of PEHs. Surgeons must recognize the role of tension and when identified attempt to lessen both axial tension along the length of the esophagus and/or radial tension pulling on the diaphragmatic closure.

Even if radiologic recurrence is an objective outcome, it seems to have little correlation with the presence of symptoms or need for surgical revision particularly when less than 2 cm in size.[13,18,19,50] In analysis of 8 different symptoms (dysphagia, heartburn, regurgitation, chest/abdominal pain, postprandial bloating, aspiration, shortness of breath, and use of PPIs) and the presence of radiographic recurrence, none of the 8 symptoms proved to be associated with the

recurrence.[15] Comparatively, others studies have suggested that new-onset dysphagia is 1 symptom that occurs more frequently[11] and is also commonly seen in patients undergoing revision.[51] Lastly, the presence of a recurrence does not seem to have an impact on patient quality of life.[11]

Resumption of Antireflux Medication

Resumption of antireflux medication is a frequently cited outcome but, in the absence of a postrepair pH test, its importance has been called into question. It is believed to represent a subjective sign of recurrent GERD symptoms, but the ubiquitous availability of these medications and their use in virtually any upper GI symptom limits the utility of this outcome. Nevertheless, between 10% and 45% of patients need antireflux medication in the first 5 years after repair.[6,13,14,17–19] Although pH testing was not completed in these studies, many patients improved when the PPIs were resumed.

In the long term, the reintroduction of antireflux medication is reported between 8% and 54% without any objective measurement of acid exposure.[10,20–23,30]

Revision Surgery

Unlike resumption of PPIs, revision surgery is uncommon. In the first year after repair, there is 1% chance of requiring revision surgery.[6] In the first 5 years postoperatively, there is a rate of 2.5% to 5% redo surgery.[14–19] In the longer term, the

Table 5
Radiologic recurrence

Authors	n[a]	Median Follow-up (mo)	Mesh (%)	Collis (%)	Radiologic Recurrence (%)	
					Any	> 2 cm
Hashemi et al,[43] 2000	21	17	—	—	4	—
Wiechmann et al,[28] 2001	60	19	—	—	7	—
Khaitan et al,[46] 2002	31	25	0	0	40	—
Diaz et al,[47] 2003	116	30	5	5	32	—
Aly et al,[48] 2005	100	48	0	0	48	—
Parameswaran et al,[7] 2006	49	19	35	—	15	—
Oelschlager et al,[49] 2006	95	6	50	5	—	9 and 24
Luketich et al,[15] 2010	445	22	13	—	—	16
Oelschlager et al,[13] 2011	60	58	50	5	—	54 and 59
Zehetner et al,[64] 2011	73	12	84	40	12	—
Dallemagne et al,[11] 2011	35	99	12	—	66	—
Targarona et al,[23] 2013	43	108	16	—	46	—
Jones et al,[50] 2015	166	25	100	—	—	21

[a] Number of patients undergoing a barium swallow.

incidence of redo surgery remains low and reported to occur between 0% and 9.9%.[10,11,20–22,30] Quality of life after revision surgery is improved and comparable to patients undergoing primary repair but lower after more than one revision.[51]

PREDICTORS OF OUTCOMES

Several factors have been identified as predictors of outcomes for patients undergoing repair of a PEH. These include the following:

1. Increase in intra-abdominal pressure
   Increase in intra-abdominal pressure, particularly in the early postoperative time, increases the risk of anatomic failure by putting stress on the repair. It is strongly suggested to treat nausea, retching, and vomiting aggressively.[50,52] Abdominal trauma is also a risk factor of recurrence by increasing the intra-abdominal pressure.[50]
2. Obesity
   Obesity is an independent risk factor of recurrence of PEH after a PEH repair.[50,52,53] The combination of a PEH repair with a Roux-en-Y gastric bypass offers an effective treatment of the obesity and a symptomatic PEH, with a concurrent reduction of antireflux medical therapy and 89% of overall satisfaction at median follow-up of 35 months.[54,55] At 13 months, a combination of PEH repair with a longitudinal gastrectomy also showed a resolution of symptoms.[56]
3. Size of the hiatal hernia
   A large crural surface area (>5.6 cm^2) of the hernia increases the risk of recurrence.[57] This is likely a surrogate measure for radial

diaphragmatic tension, which is not usually objectively measured but rather clinically assessed. Attempts to find a simple measure, such as the hiatal width, did not seem to correlate with tension but the shape of the hiatus (slit, teardrop, D, or oval) did correlate with tension.[58] Tension was reduced by use of relaxing incision, but whether this translates into a reduction in recurrence remains unclear. The use of crural mesh to decrease the risk of recurrence in large crural defect has been controversial. Level I data suggest that bioabsorbable mesh does not reduce recurrence, but proponents of synthetic mesh suggest otherwise.[13,49] Currently, the need for mesh in a majority of cases, as well as the type, size, and shape of mesh, remains controversial.[31,57]

4. Atypical symptoms
   Patients who have atypical symptoms are believed at higher risk of failure compared with those who have typical symptoms. These symptoms may be secondary to establishment over time of reflexive (and relatively refractory) development of cough and changes in lung function, creating greater pressure gradients from abdomen to chest.[53] The presence of atypical symptoms is less likely to be resolved with surgical repair, leaving patients less satisfied.

OUTCOMES IN THE ELDERLY POPULATION

Because PEHs are most commonly found in elderly patients, this group deserves a few comments. Often referring physicians are reluctant to refer elderly (>70 years) or frail patients for surgical repair, fearing the risk of surgical intervention.

Table 6
Surgical outcome in elderly population

Articles	Mean Age (Range)	n	Mean Follow-up (mo)	Radiological Recurrence (%)	Redo Surgery (%)	Reintroduction of Proton Pump Inhibitor (%)	Improvement of Symptoms (%)
Merzlikin et al,[10] 2017	77	38	24	13	0	26	—
Parker et al,[59] 2017	75 (73–77)	82	11.3	5	1.2	—	—
	83 (80–86)	45	11.3	0	—	—	—
Louie et al,[5] 2011	78	58	15.6	10	0	—	81
Gangopadhyay et al,[60] 2006	(75–91)	47	18.8	27.8	—	8.3	—
Hazebroek et al,[61] 2008	76.6 (70–85)	35	43	2.9	2.9	—	46.7

Table 7
Laparoscopic versus open paraesophageal hernia repair outcomes

Articles	Approach	n	Mean Follow-up (mo)	Radiological Recurrence (%)	Redo Surgery (%)	Reintroduction of Proton Pump Inhibitor (%)	Improvement of Symptoms (%)
Lazar et al,[30] 2017	LSC	87	79	—	9.9	54	95.4
	Open	19	84	—	5.3	25	89.5
Schauer et al,[63] 1998	LSC	67	13	—	0	—	94
	Open	25	48	—	0.08	—	84
Karmali et al,[8] 2008	LSC	46	16	9	4.3	—	81[b]
	Open	47	18	9	2.1	—	85[b]
Zehetner et al,[64] 2011	LSC	73	12	12.3	3.4[a]	—	84[a]
	Open	73	16	24.7	—	—	

Abbreviation: LSC, laparoscopic.
[a] The difference between LSC and open is not specified.
[b] Satisfaction.

These patients, however, have a significant reduction in quality of life at baseline because of the hernia. This often is amplified because eating is a huge part of the social well-being of elderly patients, who often gather for meals. Several articles have specifically documented outcomes in elderly patients (**Table 6**). These studies show a very low morbidity and virtually no mortalities in these patients. The risks rise from 70 years to 80 years of age and then again above 80 years of age.[15] Fortunately, patient improvement in quality of life is significant after surgical repair.[5,59–61]

Even in long-term follow-up of greater than 5 years after PEH repair, there remains significant improvement in quality of life as measured by Quality of Life in Reflex and Dyspepsia (QOLRAD) questionnaire, modified Dakkak swallowing score (DSS), and GERD-HRQL score.[10] None of the patients needed revisional surgery, even though there were radiologic recurrences in 13%, with 26% resuming antireflux medication. Even in patients who died before their 5-year follow-up, their quality of life just prior to death from the repair remained satisfactory, suggesting that symptomatic patients who are elderly should be evaluated for repair regardless, given surgery can still offer them a significant improvement in quality of life.[10]

COMPARATIVE OUTCOMES

The standard many investigators reference remains the 93% good to excellent outcomes (free of symptoms) at a mean follow-up of 94 months.[62] These outcomes were achieved in the era of transthoracic repair, with 80% receiving a gastroplasty and 36% of patients with erosive esophagitis or stricture. In the laparoscopic era, there are only 4 comparative studies, with all comparing to an open approach (**Table 7**). These studies report symptomatic improvements ranging from 81% to 95% and a low rate of revisional surgery from 0% to 9.9%. Radiologic recurrences were similar in 1 study but were higher after open surgery, with the laparoscopic group having more liberal use of mesh and Collis gastroplasty. Only Lazar and colleagues[30] documented long-term results at 79 months and 84 months, showing similar symptomatic improvement, slightly higher rates of revision in laparoscopic surgery, and much higher rate of PPI reintroduction in the laparoscopic group.

SUMMARY

The assessment of PEH repair and reporting of outcomes is a challenging process due to a variety of factors, including surgical preferences (including use of mesh), multiple instruments to measure outcomes, and a broad symptom and sign complex produced by the herniated intra-abdominal contents. Overall clinical outcomes after repair are excellent at short-term and 5 years' assessments, but there is a lack of longer-term data. Radiologic recurrences are a key outcome and can be minimized by liberally attending to axial tension along the esophagus (with appropriate esophageal mobilization and use of gastroplasty) and radial tension on the diaphragm (with possible use of tension-relieving maneuvers with or without mesh reinforcement).

REFERENCES

1. Draaisma W, Gooszen H, Tournoij E, et al. Controversies in paraesophageal hernia repair: a review of literature. Surg Endosc 2005;19:1300–8.
2. Lidor A, Kawaji Q, Stem K, et al. Defining recurrence after paraesophageal hernia repair: correlating

symptoms and radiographic findings. Surgery 2013; 154:171–8.

3. Oelschlager B, Ma K, Soares R, et al. A broad assessment of clinical outcomes after laparoscopic antireflux surgery. Ann Surg 2012;256:87–94.

4. Allison PR. Reflux esophagitis, sliding hiatal hernia, and the anatomy of repair. Surg Gynecol Obstet 1951;92(4):419–31.

5. Louie B, Blitz M, Farivar A, et al. Repair of symptomatic giant paraesophageal hernias in elderly (>70 years) patients results and improved quality of life. J Gastrointest Surg 2011;15:386–96.

6. Luketich J, Raja S, Fernando H, et al. Laparoscopic repair of giant paraesophageal hernia: 100 consecutive cases. Ann Surg 2000;323:608–18.

7. Parameswaran R, Ali A, Velmurugan S, et al. Laparoscopic repair of large paraesophageal hiatus hernia: quality of life and durability. Surg Endosc 2006;20: 1221–4.

8. Karmali S, McFadden S, Mitchell P, et al. Primary laparoscopic and open repair of paraesophageal hernias: a comparison of short-term outcomes. Dis Esophagus 2008;21:63–8.

9. Velanovich V. The development of the GERD-HRQL symptom severity instrument. Dis Esophagus 2007; 20:130–4.

10. Merzlikin O, Louie B, Farivar A, et al. Repair of symptomatic paraesophageal hernias in elderly (>70 years) patients results in sustained quality of life at 5 years and beyond. Surg Endosc 2017;31: 3979–84.

11. Dallemagne B, Kohnen L, Perreta S, et al. Laparoscopic repair of paraesophageal hernia. Long-term follow-up reveals good clinical outcome despite high radiological recurrence rate. Ann Surg 2011; 253:291–6.

12. Revicki D, Wood M, Wiklund I, et al. Reliability and validity of the Gastrointestinal Symptom Rating Scale in patients with gastroesophageal reflux disease. Qual Life Res 1998;7:75–83.

13. Oelschlager B, Pelligrini C, Hunter J, et al. Biologic prosthesis to prevent recurrence after laparoscopic paraesophageal hernia repair: long-term follow-up from a multicenter, prospective, randomized trial. J Am Coll Surg 2011;213:461–8.

14. Pierre A, Luketich J, Fernando H, et al. Results of laparoscopic repair of giant paraesophageal hernias: 200 consecutive patients. Ann Thorac Surg 2002;74:1909–15.

15. Luketich J, Nason K, Christie N, et al. Outcomes after a decade of laparoscopic giant paraesophageal hernia repair. J Thorac Cardiovasc Surg 2010;139: 395–404, 404.e1.

16. Lidor A, Stelle K, Stem M, et al. Long-term quality of life and risk factors for recurrence after laparoscopic repair of paraesophageal hernia. JAMA Surg 2015; 150:424–31.

17. Jobe B, Aye R, Deveney C, et al. Laparoscopic management of giant type III hiatal hernia and short esophagus. Objective follow-up at three years. J Gastrointest Surg 2002;6:181–8.

18. Nason K, Luketich J, Qureshi I, et al. Laparoscopic repair of giant paraesophageal hernia results in long-term patient satisfaction and a durable repair. J Gastrointest Surg 2008;12:2066–75.

19. Oelschlager B, Petersen R, Brunt L, et al. Laparoscopic paraesophageal hernia repair: defining long-term clinical and anatomic outcomes. J Gastrointest Surg 2012; 16:453–9.

20. Gryska P, Vernon J. Tension-free repair of hiatal hernia during laparoscopic fundoplication: a ten-year experience. Hernia 2005;9:150–5.

21. Simorov A, Ranade A, Jones R, et al. Long-term patient outcomes after laparoscopic anti-reflux procedures. J Gastrointest Surg 2014;18:157–62.

22. Lafullarde T, Watson D, Jamieson G, et al. Laparoscopic Nissen fundoplication: five-year results and beyond. Arch Surg 2001;132:180–4.

23. Targarona E, Grisales S, Uyanik O, et al. Long-term outcome and quality of life after laparoscopic treatment of large paraesophageal hernia. World J Surg 2013;37:1878–82.

24. White B, Jeansonne L, Morgenthal C, et al. Do recurrences after paraesophageal hernia repair matter? Ten-year follow-up after laparoscopic repair. Surg Endosc 2008;22:1107–11.

25. Levy G, Aye R, Farivar A, et al. A combined Nissen plus hill hybrid repair for paraesophageal hernia improves clinical outcomes and reduced long-term recurrences compared with laparoscopic Nissen alone. J Gastrointest Surg 2017;21:121–5.

26. Thompson S, Jamieson G, Myers J, et al. Recurrent heartburn after laparoscopic fundoplication is not always recurrent reflux. J Gastrointest Surg 2007;11: 642–7.

27. Granderath F. Laparoscopic Nissen fundoplication with prosthetic hiatal closure reduces postoperative intrathoracic wrap herniation: preliminary results of a prospective randomized functional and clinical study. Arch Surg 2005;140:40–8.

28. Wiechmann R, Ferguson M, Naunheim K, et al. Laparoscopic management of giant paraesophageal herniation. Ann Thorac Surg 2001;7:1080–6.

29. Mittal S, Bikhchandani J, Gurney O, et al. Outcomes after repair of the intrathoracic stomach: objective follow-up of up to 5 years. Surg Endosc 2011;25: 556–66.

30. Lazar D, Birkett D, Brams D, et al. Long-term patient-reported outcomes of paraesophageal hernia repair. JSLS 2017;21. e2017.00052.

31. Soricelli E, Basso N, Genco A, et al. Long-term results of hiatal hernia mesh repair and antireflux laparoscopic surgery. Surg Endosc 2009;23: 2499–504.

32. Aye R, Rehse D, Blitz M, et al. The Hill antireflux repair at 5 institutions over 25 years. Am J Surg 2011;201:599–604.

33. Robinson B, Dunst C, Cassera M, et al. 20 years later: laparoscopic fundoplication durability. Surg Endosc 2015;29:2520–4.

34. Senyk J, Arborelius M, Lilja B, et al. Respiratory function on esophageal hiatus. Respiration 1975; 32:93–102.

35. Low D, Simchuck. Effect of paraesophageal hernia repair on pulmonary function. Ann Thorac Surg 2002;74:333–7.

36. Segal HL. Secondary anemia associated with diaphragmatic hernia. New York State Journal of Medicine 1931;31:692–5.

37. Carrott P, Markar S, Hong J, et al. Iron-deficience anemia is a common presenting issue with giant paraesophageal nernia and resolves following repair. J Gastrointest Surg 2013;17:858–62.

38. Haurani C, Carlin A, Hammoud Z, et al. Prevalence and resolution of anemia with paraesophageal hernia repair. J Gastrointest Surg 2012;16:1817–20.

39. Hayden J, Jamieson G. Effect on iron deficiency anemia of laparoscopic repair of large paresophageal hernias. Dis Esophagus 2005;18:329–31.

40. Trastek V, Allen M, Deschamps C, et al. Diaphragmatic hernia and associated anemia: response to surgical treatment. J Thorac Cardiovasc Surg 1996;12:1340–5.

41. Windsor C, Collis J. Anaemia and hiatus hernia: experience in 450 patients. Thorax 1967;22:73–8.

42. Carrott P, Hong J, Kuppusamy M, et al. Repair of giant paraesophageal hernias routinely produces improvement in respiratory function. J Thorac Cardiovasc Surg 2012;143:398–404.

43. Hashemi M, Peters J, DeMeester T, et al. Laparoscopic repair of large type III hiatal hernia: Objective follow up reveals high recurrence rate. J Am Coll Surg 2000;190:553–60.

44. Mittal S, Shah P. Current readings: failed hiatal hernia repair. Semin Thorac Cardiovasc Surg 2014;26: 331–4.

45. Zehetner J, DeMeester S, Ayazi S, et al. Tension-free repair of hiatal hernia during laparoscopic fundoplication: a ten-year experience. Surg Endosc 2011; 22:1219–26.

46. Khaitan L, Houston H, Sharp K, et al. Laparoscopic paraesophageal hernia repair has an acceptable reucrrence rate. Am Surg 2002;68:546–52.

47. Diaz S, Brunt L, Klingensmith M, et al. Laparoscopic paraesophageal hernia repair, a challenging operation: medium term-outcome in 116 patients. J Gastrointest Surg 2003;7:59–66.

48. Aly A, Munt J, Jamieson G, et al. Laparoscopic repair of large hiatal hernias. Br J Surg 2005;92:648–53.

49. Oelschlager BK, Pellegrini CA, Hunter J, et al. Biologic prosthesis reduces recurrence after laparoscopic paraesophageal hernia repair: a multicenter, prospective, randomized trial. Ann Surg 2006;244:481–90.

50. Jones R, Simorov A, Lomelin D, et al. Long-term outcomes of radiologic recurrence after paraesophageal hernia repair with mesh. Surg Endosc 2015; 29:425–30.

51. Wilshire C, Louie B, Shultz D, et al. Clinical outcomes of reoperation for failed antireflux operation. Ann Thorac Surg 2016;101:1290–6.

52. Kohn G, Price R, DeMeester S, et al. Guidelines for the management of hiatal hernia. Surg Endosc 2013; 27:4409–28.

53. Morgenthal C, Lin E, Shane M, et al. Who will fail laparoscopic Nissen fundoplication? Preoperative prediction of long-term outcomes. Surg Endosc 2007;21:1978–84.

54. Chaudhry U, Marr B, Osayi S, et al. Laparoscopic Roux-en-Y gastric bypass for treatment of symptomatic paraesophageal hernia in the morbidly obese: medium-term results. Surg Obes Relat Dis 2014; 10:1063–7.

55. Awais O, Luketich J, Reddy N, et al. Roux-en-Y near esophagojujunostomy for failed antireflux operations: outcomes in more than 100 patients. Ann Thorac Surg 2014;98:1905–13.

56. Rodriguez J, Kroh M, El-Hayek, et al. Combined paraesophageal hernia repair and partial longitudinal gastrectomy in obese patients with symptomatic paraesophageal hernias. Surg Endosc 2012;26: 3382–90.

57. Koch O, Ashe K, Berger J, et al. Influence of the size of the hiatus on the rate of reherniation after laparoscopic fundoplication and refundopilication with mesh hiatoplasty. Surg Endosc 2011;24:1024–30.

58. Bradley D, Louie B, Farivar A, et al. Assessment and reduction of diaphragmatic tension during hiatal hernia repair. Surg Endosc 2015;29:796–804.

59. Parker D, Rambhajan A, Horsley, et al. Laparoscopic paraesophageal hernia repair is safe in elderly patients. Surg Endosc 2017;31:1186–91.

60. Gangopadhyay N, Pettone J, Sopper N, et al. Outcomes of laparoscopic paraesophageal hernia repair in elderly and high-risk patient. Surgery 2006;140:491–9.

61. Hazebroek E, Gananadha S, Koak Y, et al. Laparoscopic paraesophageal hernia repair : quality of life outcomes in the eldery. Dis Esophagus 2008;21:737–41.

62. Maziak D, Todd T, Pearson F. Massive hiatus hernia: evaluation and surgical management. Thorac Cardiovasc Surg 1998;115:53–62.

63. Schauer P, Ikramuddin S, McLughlin R, et al. Comparison of laparoscopic versus open repair of paraesophageal hernia. Am J Surg 1998;176:659–65.

64. Zehetner J, DeMeester S, Ayazi S, et al. Laparoscopic versus open repair for paraesophageal hernia: the second decade. J Am Coll Surg 2011;212:813–20.

Preoperative Evaluation and Clinical Decision Making for Giant Paraesophageal Hernias
Who Gets an Operation?

Sarah Choi, MD, Andrew Tang, MD, Sudish Murthy, MD, PhD,
Siva Raja, MD, PhD*

KEYWORDS

- Giant paraesophageal hernia • Evaluation • Volvulus • Complications • Elective operation
- Emergent operation

KEY POINTS

- Giant paraesophageal hernias can range from an asymptomatic incidentally detected paraesophageal hernia to an emergent gastric volvulus with concern for ischemia.
- Preoperative testing evaluates the gastroesophageal anatomy and function to determine the optimal operation.
- Asymptomatic patients should be counseled in regards to the risk–benefit profile of definitive repair versus observation.

INTRODUCTION

A hiatal hernia is a protrusion of the abdominal viscera from the abdominal cavity into the thoracic cavity through the esophageal hiatus of the diaphragm. Two theories of the etiology of hiatal hernias exist. One suggests that acid-induced esophageal mucosal injury (eg, gastroesophageal reflux disease) causes scarring, thus shortening and pulling the gastroesophageal junction (GEJ) superiorly toward the thoracic cavity.[1] The other suggests that the repetitive stress of swallowing or vomiting combined with increased intra-abdominal pressure (eg, pregnancy, chronic constipation, chronic obstructive pulmonary disease, obesity) leads to a weakened phrenoesophageal membrane and widening of the diaphragmatic hiatus, allowing visceral herniation to occur.[2]

Hiatal hernias are classified into 4 types (I–IV).[3] Type I is a sliding hiatal hernia that is characterized by the displacement of the GEJ into the mediastinum through the hiatus. A type II hernia is characterized by the herniation of the gastric fundus through the hiatus, while the GEJ remains fixed in the normal anatomic location, caudad to the hiatus. A type III hernia, also called a mixed type owing to its features of both type I and type II hernias, is characterized by both the GEJ and the fundus of the stomach herniating through the hiatus. Last, a type IV hernia is characterized by herniation of not only the stomach, but also intra-abdominal viscera (such as the colon, spleen, pancreas, liver, or small bowel) displaced into the chest.

Nearly 90% to 95% of hiatal hernias are estimated to be sliding hernias (type I), and 5% to

Disclosure Statement: S. Raja is a paid consultant of Smiths-Medical. All other authors have no disclosures.
Department of Thoracic and Cardiovascular Surgery, Cleveland Clinic, 9500 Euclid Avenue, Cleveland, OH 44195, USA
* Corresponding author. Department of Thoracic and Cardiovascular Surgery, Cleveland Clinic, 9500 Euclid Avenue, Desk J4-133, Cleveland, OH 44195.
E-mail address: rajas@ccf.org

Thorac Surg Clin 29 (2019) 415–419
https://doi.org/10.1016/j.thorsurg.2019.07.006
1547-4127/19/© 2019 Elsevier Inc. All rights reserved.

10% are estimated to be paraesophageal hernias (PEH; types II–IV). Among the nonsliding PEH, 90% are type III hernias.[4] Although a uniform definition does not exist across the literature, a giant hiatal hernia is a term generally used to describe hernias (usually types III and IV) with more than one-third of the stomach herniating into the chest and is a diagnosis that generally requires surgical repair.[5]

CLINICAL PRESENTATION

PEH present in a variety of ways, depending on the extent of herniation. It is estimated that up to 50% of patients with PEH are asymptomatic.[6] Symptoms from PEH can be classified as either obstructive or nonobstructive. Patients with PEH can present with dysphagia, regurgitation, epigastric pain, early satiety, postprandial fullness, nausea, emesis, and bloating secondary to a mechanical obstruction. These symptoms are more concerning for subsequent volvulus. Nonobstructive symptoms include gastroesophageal reflux and erosive esophagitis, owing to the loss of a functional lower esophageal sphincter and, chronic anemia from mucosal ulcerations (Cameron lesions). Shortness of breath is an atypical symptom that may prompt referral. The relationship to the hernia is somewhat nebulous, but there might be compressive atelectasis and shunting if a large hernia exists. Reflux-related lung injury also might conspire in this setting. However, if during a workup for dyspnea there is little compressive atelectasis or interstitial lung disease noted on a computed tomography scan of the chest, it would be difficult to connect the hernia with the pulmonary complaint.

Acute complications of gastric volvulus from PEH, including incarceration and strangulation, require urgent surgical evaluation owing to the risk of ischemia, perforation, and necrosis. Patients with acute gastric volvulus may present with Borchardt's triad of symptoms: (1) severe epigastric pain, (2) retching with an inability to vomit, and (3) an inability to pass a nasogastric tube into the stomach.[7] This condition is a true surgical emergency.

INDICATIONS FOR SURGERY

Historically, PEHs were repaired when identified, regardless of symptoms. This practice stems from studies published by Belsey and Hill, which showed up to a 29% mortality rate if presenting with acute volvulus.[8,9] However, recent studies have shown a lower frequency of complications, as low as 1.1% per year for asymptomatic or mildly symptomatic PEHs managed with careful surveillance.[10] Only 0.9% of patients admitted and treated for PEH from 1998 to 2008 had gangrenous complications from acute volvulus.[11] As such, surgical decision making should be based on symptoms rather than a historical fear of gastric necrosis.

The decision to operate on PEHs in the elective setting largely depends on whether a patient is symptomatic. Patients with symptomatic PEH should undergo a definitive surgical repair unless comorbidities are prohibitive. All asymptomatic patients should have a discussion with a foregut surgeon for elective repair versus observation, taking into consideration the patient's age and comorbidities as well as the size of the PEH.

An emergent operation is indicated for acute complications from gastric volvulus of PEHs such as incarceration, strangulation, or perforation.

PREOPERATIVE EVALUATION

Preoperative studies to evaluate PEHs should include an upper gastrointestinal (UGI) series, esophagogastroduodenoscopy (EGD), a computed tomography scan of the abdomen and pelvis with contrast for patients with prior history of abdominal or esophageal surgery, a 4-hour gastric emptying study in patients without esophageal obstruction, esophageal high-resolution manometry (HRM), and cardiopulmonary testing (eg, pulmonary function tests, cardiac stress tests). These diagnostic tests provide valuable information regarding the anatomy and help to rule out other etiologies that may explain symptoms. These tests also help to determine the appropriate operative approach.

An UGI series is usually the best initial test to help identify the size and anatomic location of the esophagus and stomach, specifically the position of the GEJ and its relation to the esophageal hiatus.[12] It also helps to identify the axis of volvulus. Organoaxial voluvus, which is most common, occurs when the stomach rotates around the cardia–pylorus longitudinal axis (**Fig. 1**). Mesoenteric volvulus, which is much rarer, occurs when the stomach rotates perpendicular to the cardio–pylorus longitudinal axis.[13] This contrast study also provides information of gastric outlet or esophageal obstruction should it exist. It may also identify a short esophagus, which would allow the surgeon to plan for an esophageal lengthening procedure, such as a Collis gastroplasty.[14]

An EGD should be performed on all patients with suspected PEH. It allows for direct visualization of the mucosa and helps to define the anatomy and size of a hernia. The nonreducible component of PEHs are usually identified by retroflexion of the

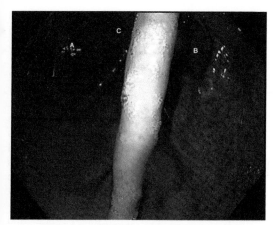

Fig. 1. EGD demonstrating organoaxial volvulus. (A) Gastric inlet. (B) Gastric outlet. (C) Endoscope on retroflexion.

scope. The diagnosis can also be made by identifying the GEJ in relation to the diaphragmatic pinch, which is the indentation on the stomach from the diaphragmatic hiatus. A separate orifice adjacent to the GEJ on retroflexion, containing gastric rugal folds, indicates a type II hernia, whereas gastric rugal folds noted above the diaphragm with the GEJ entering midway up the pouch indicates a type III hernia.[14] An EGD also helps to rule out other abnormal pathology such as Barrett's esophagus, esophagitis, stricture, and esophageal or gastric cancer before PEH repair.

A 4-hour gastric emptying study may be useful for patients with symptoms of delayed gastric emptying such as nausea, vomiting, postprandial fullness, early satiety, and bloating. In a subset of patients with delayed gastric emptying, an additional emptying procedure such as botulinum toxin (Botox) to the pylorus or pyloromyotomy may be done intraoperatively. We do not routinely advocate a pyloroplasty in patients with delayed gastric emptying because these symptoms could be due to the volvulus or a highly dysfunctional GEJ sphincter mechanism; however, patients with a higher risk of gastric dysmotility secondary to dysautonomia (diabetic neuropathy, primary dysautonomias, etc), neurologic disorders (multiple sclerosis, Parkinson disease, etc), infiltrative diseases (scleroderma, amyloidosis, etc), and previous foregut operations, may benefit from an additional emptying procedure.

The last test to define the anatomy of the hernia is the abdominal and pelvic computed tomography scan in patients with prior abdominal or esophageal surgery. Although this procedure allows the surgeon to differentiate between a type III and type IV hernia based on the viscera in the hernia sac, it often does not change the surgical plan. However, in patients with prior surgery, it can be important to establish their preoperative anatomy to plan an approach from the abdomen or chest.

HRM can provide valuable information regarding the lower esophageal sphincter location and function (to rule out achalasia) and, more important, allows for the assessment of esophageal motility, especially in patients with a dilated esophagus on a UGI series. The need for HRM is controversial and debated among surgeons; however, in our opinion, it is helpful for patients whose main symptoms are dysphagia, because it helps to determine the appropriate operative approach. With findings of aperistalsis or dysmotility on HRM, a partial (Toupet vs Dor) or no fundoplication (instead of a Nissen fundoplication) might be indicated. However, depending on the tortuosity of the hernia, accurate placement of the manometry catheter can prove very challenging.

The use of a pH test is controversial. We do not find it changes our operation when used preoperatively, but it is a useful tool postoperatively, after the anatomy has been corrected, to determine which patients need to continue antacid medications.

Once the hernia anatomy and esophageal function have been delineated, the perioperative risk should be determined. A general cardiopulmonary assessment, including a chest radiograph and electrocardiogram will help to determine if a patient can tolerate general anesthesia. For patients who present with shortness of breath or chest pain, it would be prudent to obtain pulmonary function tests to rule out underlying pulmonary disease as the cause of shortness of breath and an echocardiogram to rule out cardiac dysfunction as the culprit of symptoms. Patients who present with chest pain may also benefit from a cardiac stress test to rule out myocardial ischemia as the source of chest pain.

DECISION-MAKING ALGORITHM

There are no clear guidelines regarding management of giant PEH. General guidelines for management of hiatal hernias exist, but are highly variable depending on surgeon and institutional preferences. We offer an algorithm (**Fig. 2**) that may guide others in ordering appropriate preoperative studies, which are crucial for determining the proper operative approach for treating giant PEH.

In an acute setting, fluid resuscitation and nasogastric tube decompression are the initial steps in an evaluation. Time to operation depends on the patient's clinical stability. In patients who are

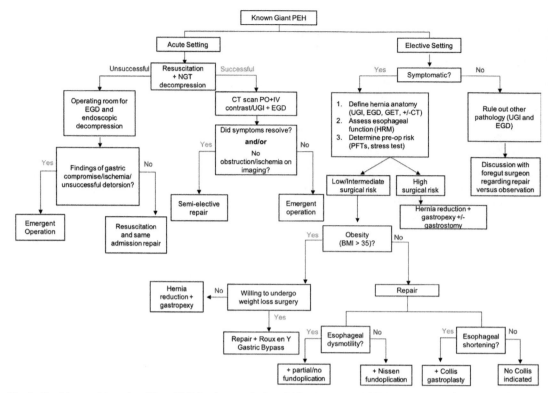

Fig. 2. Decision making algorithm. BMI, body mass index; IV, intravenous; NGT, nasogastric tube; PFTs, pulmonary function test; PO, oral.

refractory to resuscitation or cannot be adequately decompressed with a nasogastric tube, operative endoscopy is indicated. Endoscopy is diagnostic and potentially therapeutic in this case. An operative EGD will help to determine if there is mucosal necrosis and it allows for endoscopic decompression and possible detorsion. If mucosal necrosis is present or decompression is unsuccessful, then this would necessitate emergent operation. If decompression and resuscitation are successful, then same admission repair would be indicated. If patients are initially decompressed and their symptoms recur or they again become obstructed during the resuscitation period, an then emergent operation would be required. The extent of the operation is dictated by the presence of gastric necrosis, tissue edema, and clinical stability at the time of operation.

In an elective setting, preoperative evaluation depends on whether a patient is symptomatic or not. In asymptomatic patients, abnormal pathology should be ruled out using the UGI series and EGD. The surgeon should counsel the patient on the risk-benefit profile of pursuing a repair versus careful observation.

In symptomatic patients, operative repair of PEH is indicated and the previously described

preoperative tests should be ordered. In low and intermediate surgical risk patients, PEH repair is indicated. Obesity is a risk factor for hernia recurrence after PEH repair; therefore, to definitively fix the PEH, obese patients with a body mass index (BMI) of greater than or equal to 35 should consider undergoing a Roux-en-Y gastric bypass at the time of their repair.[12] Sleeve gastrectomy should be avoided, because of the increased risk of acid reflux after sleeve gastrectomy.[15] For obese patients (BMI of ≥35), who either do not qualify or refuse to undergo Roux-en-Y gastric bypass, we recommend hernia reduction with gastropexy until sufficient weight loss can be achieved for definitive repair. For patients with a BMI of less than 35, a repair without weight loss surgery is indicated. However, patients with a BMI between 25 and 35 should lose weight through medical or lifestyle modifications to decrease the risk of hernia recurrence. Whether or not a partial or complete fundoplication or an esophageal lengthening procedure (such as a Collis gastroplasty) is necessary is determined by the preoperative evaluation of anatomy and esophageal function. In high surgical risk patients, reduction of hernia and abdominal contents with a gastropexy can prevent future complications while mitigating surgical risk.

SUMMARY

Giant PEH can present in a variety of ways, ranging from an asymptomatic, incidentally detected PEH to an emergent gastric volvulus with concern for ischemia. Through thoughtful preoperative evaluation, the best operative approach can be tailored to each patient.

REFERENCES

1. Patterson W, Kolyn D. Esophageal shortening induced by short-term intraluminal acid perfusion in opossum: a cause for hiatus hernia? Gastroenterology 1994;107(6):1736–40.
2. Kahrilas PJ, Wu S, Lin S, et al. Attenuation of esophageal shortening during peristalsis with hiatus hernia. Gastroenterology 1995;109(6):1818–25.
3. Ackerland A, Onnell H, Key E. Hernia diaphragmatica hiatus oesophagei vom anastomischen und roentgenologischen gesichtspunkt. Acta Radiol 1926;6:3–22.
4. Kahrilas PJ, Kim HC, Pandolfino JE. Approaches to the diagnosis and grading of hiatal hernia. Best Pract Res Clin Gastroenterol 2008;22(4):601–16.
5. Mitiek MO, Andrade RS. Giant hiatal hernia. Ann Thorac Surg 2010;89(6):S2168–73.
6. Schieman C, Grondin SC. Paraesophageal hernia: clinical presentation, evaluation, and management controversies. Thorac Surg Clin 2009;19(4):473–84.
7. Auyang E, Oelschlager B. Laparoscopic repair of paraesophageal hernias. In: Swanstrom L, Soper N, editors. Mastery of endoscopic and laparoscopic surgery. Philadelphia: Lippincott Williams & Wilkins; 2013.
8. Hill LD. Incarcerated paraesophageal hernia: a surgical emergency. Am J Surg 1973;126(2):286–91.
9. Skinner D, Belsey R. Surgical management of esophageal reflux and hiatal hernia: long-term results with 1030 patients. J Thorac Cardiovasc Surg 1967;53:33–54.
10. Stylopoulos N, Gazelle GS, Rattner DW. Paraesophageal hernias: operation or observation? Ann Surg 2002;236(4):492–501.
11. Paul S, Mirza FM, Nasar A, et al. Prevalence, outcomes, and a risk-benefit analysis of diaphragmatic hernia admissions: an examination of the National Inpatient Sample database. J Thorac Cardiovasc Surg 2011;142(4):747–54.
12. Mittal SK, DeMeester SR, Stefanidis D, et al. Guidelines for the management of hiatal hernia. Surg Endosc 2013;27(12):4409–28.
13. Baker ME, Rice TW. Radiologic evaluation of the esophagus: methods and value in motility disorders and GERD. Semin Thorac Cardiovasc Surg 2001;13(3):201–25.
14. Dickason TJ, Lerner C, Mittal SK, et al. The preoperative predictability of the short esophagus in patients with stricture or paraesophageal hernia. Surg Endosc 2002;14(5):464–8.
15. Sweeney JF, Lin E, Urrego HD, et al. Association of radiographic morphology with early gastroesophageal reflux disease and satiety control after sleeve gastrectomy. J Am Coll Surg 2014;219(3):430–8.

Common Tenets in Repair of Primary Paraesophageal Hernias
Reducing Tension and Maximizing Length

Ankit Dhamija, MD[a], Jeremiah A. Hayanga, MD[a], Kamil A. Abbas[b], Ghulam Abbas, MD, MHCM[c],*

KEYWORDS

- Giant paraesophageal hernia • Tension-free repair • Principles

KEY POINTS

- Tension-free repair of giant paraesophageal hernia decreases the risk of recurrence.
- Axial tension is reduced by extensive circumferential esophageal dissection and mobilization. An esophageal lengthening procedure may be necessary for a short esophagus.
- Radial tension is decreased by crural dissection and mobilization. Adjunctive procedures such as pleurotomy or diaphragmatic relaxation incision may be needed.

The first report of elective hiatal hernia repair was published by Angelo Soresi in 1919.[1] As interest grew, the Mayo group published their experience with 27 patients in 1928.[2] Appreciation of hiatal hernia as a significant clinical problem coincided with the adoption of X-ray imaging.[3] Increasing radiologic diagnosis led to a rising interest in surgical repair and the rapid development of a variety of surgical techniques in the first half of the twentieth century. Rudolph Nissen, in New York Maimonides and subsequently in Switzerland, continued to focus on an abdominal approach for the repair of hiatal hernias with fundoplication.[4,5] Richard Sweet described his transthoracic technique in 1950, citing the use of principles developed from the repair of inguinal hernias. He later reported his experience in more than 100 patients with acceptable outcomes.[6,7] During the same era, Philip Allison and Norman Barrett further advanced the techniques of the surgical repair of hiatal hernia and the understanding of its association with gastroesophageal reflux.[8,9]

This work led to further advancement in the management of hiatal hernias during the second half of the twentieth century. The initial focus was on the anatomic correction of the hiatal hernia with the hope that it would also alleviate the reflux symptoms. Since then, the focus of modern surgical approaches has taken into account the combination of 2 basic concepts; first, the anatomic correction of the hiatal hernia; and second, the fundoplication or restoration of the angle of His. These concepts were the basis of further advancement of techniques by Belsey, Skinner, and Hill. Almost all the pioneers emphasized the importance of reducing the hiatal hernia, providing adequate esophageal length below the diaphragm and performing a tension-free repair.

BASIC PRINCIPLES OF HIATAL HERNIA REPAIR

The high recurrence rate associated with the repair of the larger hiatal hernia continues to be a challenge. In 1973, Allison presented the long-term

Disclosure Statement: The authors have nothing to disclose.
[a] Department of Cardiovascular and Thoracic Surgery, WVU Medicine, 1 Medical Center Drive, Morgantown, WV 26506, USA; [b] West Virginia University Honors College, 1 Medical Center Drive, Morgantown, WV 26506, USA; [c] Division of Thoracic Surgery, WVU Medicine, 1 Medical Center Drive, Morgantown, WV 26506, USA
* Corresponding author.
E-mail address: ghulam.abbas@hsc.wvu.edu

follow-up of his series on giant paraesophageal hernia and reported a 49% recurrence rate.[10] Most clinicians believe that recurrence is due to increased tension on the repair.

The 2 basic principles of tension-free hiatal hernia repair are to reduce the following:

1. Axial tension, which is assessed by adequate intra-abdominal esophageal length, which is optimized by mediastinal dissection or by additionally performing an esophageal lengthening procedure such as a Collis gastroplasty.
2. Radial tension, which is reduced by producing a tension-free diaphragmatic crural repair.

MAXIMIZING THE LENGTH AND REDUCING THE AXIAL TENSION

The necessity of a good mediastinal dissection in repair of a paraesophageal hernia cannot be overemphasized. Irrespective of the approach, the hernia sac must be dissected with complete mobilization of the esophagus up to the subcarinal level in order to attain maximum natural esophageal length. The authors almost always use a laparoscopic or robotic approach for the repair of even giant paraesopahgeal hernias. The hernia sac is manipulated at the highest point in the mediastinum and pulled caudad to the level of hiatus, and the dissection is performed using the energy device. Alternatively, the dissection of the sac may be started adjacent to the right crus. Subsequently, all paraesophageal attachments are incised. The esophagus is elevated and retroesophageal dissection is performed up to the subcarinal level, mobilizing the esophagus off the descending aorta (**Fig. 1**). The higher mediastinal dissection should be performed carefully and under direct vision so as to avoid injury of critical structures such as the airway, the aorta, and the heart. At this point the gastroesophageal junction and its relation to the left crus is identified. It is recommended to have 2 to 3 cm of esophageal length

below the hiatus for fundoplication. The best way to confirm the intra-abdominal esophageal length is to mobilize the fat pad off the gastroesophageal junction to identify the angle of His. Subsequently the left and right crura are held together with a grasper and the length of intra-abdominal esophagus is judged posteriorly. If the length is less than 2 cm, an esophageal lengthening procedure, such as Collis gastroplasty, should be considered. In recent literature, a Collis gastroplasty has been described to be essential in 3% to 4% of patients.[11,12] In the authors' experience, almost 5% of patients with giant paraesophageal hernias would need an esophageal lengthening procedure. The authors perform laparoscopic/robotic wedge gastroplasty as the preferred esophageal lengthening procedure as described by Terry and colleagues.[13] In the authors' experience, the outcomes of robotic versus laparoscopic repair of giant paraesophageal hernia are comparable except when it is necessary to perform an esophageal lengthening procedure. The authors find the robotic approach for wedge gastroplasty superior to the laparoscopic approach because the use of robotic staplers makes the procedure easier and more efficient.

TENSION-FREE DIAPHRAGMATIC CRURAL REPAIR: MANAGING THE RADIAL TENSION

Radial tension is directed as perpendicular to the long axis of the esophagus, parallel to the diaphragmatic crura and away from the midline. Reduction of this tension is required to help reestablish the antireflux mechanism of the lower esophageal sphincter, and assists in reapproximating the hiatus.

In most cases this can be achieved by meticulous hiatal dissection. However, certain situations may require an adjunctive procedure to decrease the tension on the crural repair. Historically, some surgeons advocated temporary phrenic nerve manipulation causing elevation of the diaphragm and reduction of tension. For example, Harrington[2] discussed creating a cervical incision and neurolyzing the phrenic nerve to paralyze the left hemidiaphragm and decrease the tension on the repair. Sweet[6] also described crushing the phrenic nerve as part of his transthoracic repair of hiatal hernia.

In this laparoscopic/robotic era, however, the following steps facilitate tension-free repair and crural approximation during primary closure.

Meticulous Crural Dissection

This component includes dissection of crura both on their outer and inner surfaces. The

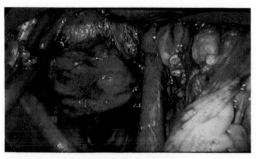

Fig. 1. Post–mediastinal dissection view of the mediastinum showing circumferential mobilization of the esophagus to the level of subcarina.

gastrohepatic ligament is incised along the right crus, then the fibrous attachments at the outer surface of the apex of the right crus are incised up to the phrenic vein. At the apex, the plane between the hernia sac and the inner aspect of the right crus is entered. Subsequently, retroesophageal dissection is performed to expose the decussation of the right and left crural fiber at the base. This area is cleared and attachments to the posterior surface of the esophagus are incised. At this point, the layer of fibrous tissue, which is found just on the inner surface of the left crus and attached to the esophagus, is incised (**Fig. 2**). This is an important step in achieving mobilization of the left crus. The next step is to dissect the base of left crus. The surgeon best performs this by passing the left-hand instrument behind the esophagus and pulling the left crus to the right while the assistant elevates the esophagus to provide retraction. The energy device on the surgeon's right hand will dissect the soft tissue off the base of the left crus. Later, once the short gastric vessels are incised, the fundus will be pulled to the right, exposing the base of the left crus from the splenic side. Further dissection of the outer surface of the left crus is performed from this angle, and splenic attachments to the left crus are incised (**Fig. 3**), thus enabling complete mobilization of the left crus.

The best way to gauge the amount of tension on the repair is by haptic feel and visual clues. When the repair is under tension, certain adjunctive procedures can help to reduce the tension. One simple method to decrease tension is to create a left pleurotomy if not already done during mediastinal dissection. This leads to an increase in intrathoracic pressure and pushes the left hemidiaphragm down, making it easier to approximate the crura.

Diaphragmatic relaxation incisions on the right or left, or both sides, can also be created, if needed, to achieve a tension-free repair. Greene and colleagues[14] prefer a right-sided relaxation

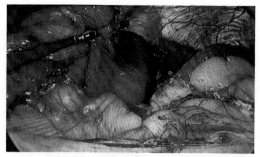

Fig. 3. Dissection and mobilization of the left crus base, including mobilization of the splenic attachments to the diaphragm.

incision. They recommend an ipsilateral pleurotomy followed by an incision parallel to inferior vena cava, leaving a 3- to 5-mm tissue cuff along the vena cava for suturing the patch. This extends from the midportion of the right crus and ends below the anterior crural vein. Posterior extension of the incision is not recommended because there is usually not much tension at the base of crus and, moreover, posterior extension risks thoracic duct injury. The gap is closed using a synthetic patch. By contrast, a left-sided relaxing incision tends to be longer and bigger than the right, beginning to the left of the hiatus, and follows the course of the seventh rib laterally, salvaging a 1- to 2-cm cuff of diaphragm to sew to. The course is parallel to the rib and is not a radial incision, so as to avoid injury to the left phrenic nerve and subsequent paralysis of the left hemidiaphragm. The defect is then repaired with a 1-mm thick polytetrafluoroethylene (PTFE) patch. On the right, usually the patch required is smaller and sewn in place with interrupted sutures, whereas a larger patch is needed on the left because of a larger post–relaxation incision defect (**Fig. 4**).

The use of the falciform ligament as hiatal reinforcement or hiatal bridging has also been described in the literature. Laird and colleagues[15] described the falciform ligament mostly being used to reinforce the hiatal closure, and in their series of 33 patients 3 had radiographic recurrence, with only one being symptomatic. Park and colleagues[16] used the falciform ligament as an autologous tissue to bridge the hiatus, with no patients requiring postoperative interventions related to the hiatal hernia repair.

The use of both synthetic and biological mesh for crural reinforcement is also well described in the literature. Frantzides and colleagues[17] showed zero recurrence in the patients who underwent reinforcement of crural repair with PTFE mesh compared with 22% recurrence in the group that

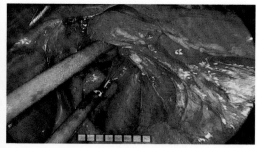

Fig. 2. The fibrous attachments on the inner surface of the left crus.

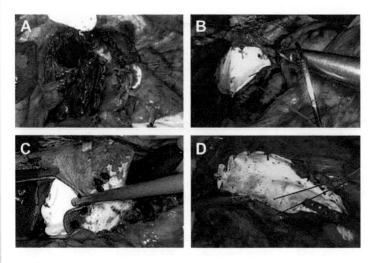

Fig. 4. (*A*) After a right relaxing incision, the hiatus is closed tidily with minimal tension. (*B*) The defect is closed with 1-mm PTFE mesh. (*C*) The primary crural closure is reinforced with an absorbable mesh that also covers the PTFE patch. (*D*) A left relaxing incision is closed with a 1-mm PTFE patch. (*From* Greene CL, DeMeester SR, Zehetner J, et al. Diaphragmatic relaxing incisions during laparoscopic paraesophageal hernia repair. Surg Endosc 2013;27:4532–4538; with permission.)

had primary crural repair. Similarly, Granderath and colleagues[18] from Austria showed a 1% recurrence rate with the use of polypropylene mesh compared with a 6% recurrence rate in the non-mesh group. Follow-up reports associated the use of synthetic mesh with dysphagia caused by scarring and erosion into esophageal and gastric lumen, with catastrophic outcomes. Oelschlager and colleagues[19] used biological mesh for crural reinforcement. Although the recurrence rate was significantly lower at 6 months in the mesh group than in the primary repair group (9% vs 24%), there was no difference in recurrence rate or other outcomes at 5 years.

The association between the use of mesh during hiatal hernia repair and dysphagia or erosion continues to be a concern. Even biological mesh shrinks over time and undergoes scar formation, potentially causing dysphagia. The use of mesh to bridge the hiatal gap should be performed with extreme caution and is better avoided. Although it may prevent short-term recurrence, this approach potentially can lead to significant dysphagia or erosion over time owing to formation of a bridge of scar posterior to the esophagus.

SUMMARY

The minimally invasive surgical management of giant paraesophageal hernias remains challenging, with a high recurrence rate. Tension-free repair with adequate intra-abdominal esophageal length remains the key principle of a successful outcome. Adequate circumferential mediastinal dissection up to the level of the carina gives the maximum natural esophageal length and hence decreases the axial tension. An esophageal lengthening procedure should be considered for the short

esophagus. Crural dissection is necessary for tension-free approximation of the crura. Diaphragmatic relaxation incisions may be necessary if the crural repair is deemed to be under tension.

REFERENCES

1. Soresi AL. Diaphragmatic hernia: its unsuspected frequency: diagnosis and technique for radical cure. Ann Surg 1919;69:254–70.
2. Harrington SW. Diaphragmatic hernia. Arch Surg 1928;16:386–415.
3. Moore AB, Kirklin BR. Progress in the roentgenological diagnosis of diaphragmatic hernia. JAMA 1930; 95:1966–9.
4. Nissen R. Eine einfache Operation zur Beeinflussung der Refluxeosophagitis. Schweiz Med Wochenschr 1956;86:590–2.
5. Nissen R. Reminiscences: reflux esophagitis and hiatal hernia. Rev Surg 1970;27:307–14.
6. Sweet RH. Diaphragmatic hernia. In: Sweet RH, editor. Thoracic surgery. Philadelphia: WB Saunders; 1950. p. 316–34.
7. Sweet RH. Esophageal hiatus hernia of the diaphragm: anatomical characteristics, technique of repair, results of treatment in 111 consecutive cases. Ann Surg 1952;135:1–13.
8. Allison PR. Reflux esophagitis, sliding hiatal hernia and anatomy of repair. Surg Gynecol Obstet 1951; 92:419–31.
9. Barrett NR. Hiatus hernia. Br J Surg 1954;42: 231–43.
10. Allison PR. Hiatus hernia: (a 20-year retrospective survey). Ann Surg 1973;178(3):273–6.
11. Swanstrom LL, Marcus DR, Galloway GQ. Laparoscopic Collis gastroplasty is the treatment of choice for the shortened esophagus. Am J Surg 1996;171: 477–81.

12. Johnson AB, Oddsdottir M, Hunter JG. Laparoscopic Collis gastroplasty and Nissen fundoplication: a new technique for the management of esophageal foreshortening. Surg Endosc 1998;12:1055–60.

13. Terry ML, Vernon A, Hunter JG. Stapled-wedge Collis gastroplasty for the shortened esophagus. Am J Surg 2004;188:195–9.

14. Greene CL, DeMeester SR, Zehetner J, et al. Diaphragmatic relaxing incisions during laparoscopic paraesophageal hernia repair. Surg Endosc 2013; 27:4532–8.

15. Laird R, Brody F, Harr JN, et al. Laparoscopic repair of paraesophageal hernia with a falciform ligament buttress. J Gastrointest Surg 2015;19(7):1223–8.

16. Park AE, Hoogerboord CM, Sutton E. Use of the falciform ligament flap for closure of the esophageal hiatus in giant paraesophageal hernia. J Gastrointest Surg 2012;16(7):1417–21.

17. Frantzides CT, Madan AK, Carlson MA, et al. A prospective randomized trial of laparoscopic polytetrafluoroethylene (PTFE) patch repair vs simple cruroplasty for large hiatal hernia. Arch Surg 2002; 137(6):649–52.

18. Granderath FA, Schweiger UM, Kamolz T, et al. Laparoscopic Nissen fundoplication with prosthetic hiatal closure reduces postoperative intrathoracic wrap herniation: preliminary results of a prospective randomized functional and clinical study. Arch Surg 2005;140(1):40–8.

19. Oelschlager BK, Petersen RP, Brunt LM, et al. Laparoscopic paraesophageal hernia repair: defining long-term clinical and anatomic outcomes. J Gastrointest Surg 2012;16(3):453–9.

Management of Recurrent Paraesophageal Hernia

Tadeusz D. Witek, MD[a], James D. Luketich, MD[b], Arjun Pennathur, MD[a], Omar Awais, DO[c],*

KEYWORDS

- Recurrent paraesophageal hernia • Redo hiatal surgery • Esophagus • Esophageal surgery

KEY POINTS

- Recurrent paraesophageal hernias are associated with significant symptoms leading to increased complications and can pose a great challenge for even experienced esophageal surgeons.
- Before undergoing repair of recurrent PEH, patients require a comprehensive work-up. Work-up should include a thorough history and physical examination, review of prior operative notes, and appropriate diagnostic testing.
- Redo fundoplication with or without a gastroplasty, Roux-en-Y near esophagojejunostomy, or an esophagectomy are options available for recurrent paraesophageal hernia and need to be considered on an individual basis.
- Complete dissection of the hernia sac and reduction of the contents; preservation of vagus nerves and crural integrity; complete takedown of the previous repair; restoration of normal anatomy; complete mobilization of the esophagus, including mediastinal mobilization; defining the gastroesophageal junction after dissection of the gastroesophageal fat pad; and assessment of adequate intraabdominal esophageal length are critical steps during repair of recurrent paraesophageal hernia.
- Although there are many approaches to repair, a minimally invasive approach can be performed by surgeons with extensive experience in minimally invasive esophageal surgery.

INTRODUCTION

Paraesophageal hernias (PEHs) have long been described to cause not only reflux symptoms but also a constellation of mechanical and obstructive symptoms, and, if left unrepaired, can lead to significant morbidity.[1] The tenets of repair include reduction of the hernia sac, crural closure with or without mesh, addition of a possible lengthening procedure in the setting of a short esophagus, and a fundoplication. Although historically PEH repairs were approached through either a laparotomy or thoracotomy,[2] the paradigm has shifted to minimally invasive techniques. PEH are now most commonly repaired through a laparoscopic approach with comparable results.[3–8] Nonetheless, recurrent PEHs after initial repair are becoming more common and can range from 5% to 59%.[9] Factors that may contribute to failure include failure of recognizing a short esophagus, inadequate crural closure, and obesity with increase in body mass index (BMI). The most common type of hernia following primary PEH repair is a small sliding-type hernia. Small sliding hernias may be asymptomatic. Regardless of the cause, those recurrent PEHs that present with significant symptoms are associated with increased complications and can pose a great challenge for even experienced esophageal surgeons.

Disclosure: Funding disclosure: No external funds. This manuscript was supported by department funding, Department of Cardiothoracic Surgery, University of Pittsburgh Medical Center.
[a] Department of Cardiothoracic Surgery, University of Pittsburgh Medical Center, 200 Lothrop Street, Suite C-800, Pittsburgh, PA 15213, USA; [b] Department of Cardiothoracic Surgery, University of Pittsburgh Medical Center, 200 Lothrop Street, Suite C-816, Pittsburgh, PA 15213, USA; [c] Department of Cardiothoracic Surgery, University of Pittsburgh Medical Center, UPMC Mercy, 1400 Locust Street, Pittsburgh, PA 15219, USA
* Corresponding author.
E-mail address: awaiso@upmc.edu

Thorac Surg Clin 29 (2019) 427–436
https://doi.org/10.1016/j.thorsurg.2019.07.011
1547-4127/19/© 2019 Elsevier Inc. All rights reserved.

Although the rate of recurrent PEH can be high, the incidence of patients requiring repair is much lower. Many patients that have a small radiographic recurrence of their PEHs have minimal symptoms and can be observed. For patients that have mild to moderate symptoms, many can be managed with a combination of antireflux therapy and diet modification. However, the authors recommend that those that have significant or persistent symptoms, or those that have a large recurrent type II or III PEH, or any recurrent type IV PEH, undergo repair.

There are several surgical options for symptomatic patients with recurrent PEHs. Many factors are taken into consideration when determining the best surgical option (**Table 1**). These factors include number of prior redo operations, the state of the esophagus, and BMI. The surgical options include a redo fundoplication with possible addition of a Collis gastroplasty, Roux-en-Y near esophagojejunostomy (RNYNEJ), and an esophagectomy. The goal in patients with benign esophageal disease should always be esophageal preservation; however, in certain subset of patients, this is not always a viable option. There are several different approaches to repair of recurrent PEH, and these include open repairs either through a laparotomy or thoracotomy, or minimally invasive approaches through laparoscopy or thoracoscopy. Although surgical repair of a recurrent PEH is more challenging than the initial repair, recurrent PEH repairs can usually be accomplished through a laparoscopic approach by experienced esophageal surgeons and is our preferred surgical approach.

SURGICAL TECHNIQUE
Preoperative Planning

Before undergoing repair of recurrent PEH, patients usually require a comprehensive work-up. This work-up not only allows appropriate surgical planning, it may also identify potential causes that led to failure of the initial repair. Review of prior operative notes is imperative, especially if the prior operations were performed by a different surgeon. A detailed review focusing on esophageal mobilization, vagal preservation, division of the short gastric vessels, creation of a fundoplication, and crural repair (primarily or with mesh) not only provides a better understanding of the patent's current anatomy but also gives insight into the technical causes of failure of the initial repair.

A detailed and complete history and physical examination is essential in the evaluation of the patients. A detailed history as to the symptoms, response to the first operation, or medical treatment may sometimes uncover a motility disorder that may originally have been missed. Other warning signs that can be recognized during the preoperative evaluation include the presence of chronic opioid use and presence of severe constipation that has not resolved. These signs may add to the complexities for successful redo antireflux surgery. Preoperative evaluation also includes a barium esophagram and esophagogastroduodenoscopy (EGD). Patients with chronically incarcerated PEH may have anemia from ulcerations or gastritis. Blood tests including serum albumin are useful to evaluate nutritional status. A barium esophagram is simple and inexpensive but

Table 1				
Surgical options for recurrent paraesophageal hernia				
Options for Recurrent PEH	**Redo Fundoplication ± Gastroplasty**	**Roux-en-Y Near Esophagojejunostomy**	**Esophagectomy**	**Gastropexy[a]**
Factors to consider for each option	• First-time redo • Normal esophageal motility • Symptoms of reflux • Normal BMI	• Obese patient with comorbidities (eg, diabetes mellitus, hyperlipidemia, obstructive sleep apnea) • Esophageal dysmotility	• Severe esophageal dysmotility • Multiple prior redo foregut surgeries • Strictures • Symptoms of obstruction • Esophageal ischemia • High-grade dysplasia	• Unstable patients • Elderly patients with significant comorbidities and minimal reflux symptoms

[a] Further analysis of outcomes after gastropexy needs to be done for definitive recommendations.

extremely useful in defining the anatomy. EGD allows mucosal inspection, evaluation of anatomic abnormalities (eg, strictures), assessment of the location and integrity of the prior fundoplication, and assessment of the esophageal length. In instances in which patients present with a volvulized PEH, EGD allows assessment of the viability of the esophagus and stomach. Biopsies can be done to evaluate for Barrett and/or cancer. Computed tomography, esophageal manometry, pH testing, and gastric emptying studies are done selectively.

Although a redo fundoplication with or without a gastroplasty after complete reduction of the hernia contents and sac is the most common surgical method for treatment of recurrence, other options include a Roux-en-Y near esophagojejunostomy (**Fig. 1**) or an esophagectomy (**Fig. 2**). These options need to be considered before embarking on a repair of a recurrent PEH. Several factors weigh into surgical planning. Gastropexy may be considered as a last option, especially for elderly patients with many comorbidities, minimal reflux symptoms, and/or poor esophageal motility. RNYNEJ should be considered in obese patients that have other comorbidities, such as diabetes, sleep apnea, and hyperlipidemia.[10]

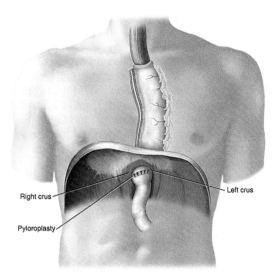

Fig. 2. Esophagectomy with reconstruction. (*From* Shah RD, Levy RM, Luketich JD. Minimally invasive Ivor Lewis esophagectomy. In: Luketich J, editor. Master techniques in surgery: esophageal surgery. Philadelphia: Wolters Kluwer Health; 2014. p. 286; with permission.)

Esophagectomy is rarely done for benign reasons such as PEH. However, it should be considered in patients that have had multiple previous foregut surgeries or patients that have evidence of a severely diseased esophagus, such as severe dysmotility, strictures, and/or significant ischemia. If an esophagectomy is being considered preoperatively, then a preoperative colonoscopy should be obtained in the event the colon is needed for a conduit. The final decision on the appropriate option is made intraoperatively after complete evaluation.

Preparation and Patient Positioning

The authors institute a standard protocol for any patient undergoing elective repair of a recurrent PEH. The patients are placed on a clear liquid diet for 2 days before the surgery. They are also given a modified bowel prep with 1 L of polyethylene glycol electrolyte solution the day before. We found that it helps compress the gastrointestinal tract to aid in dissection, and, in the event of an inadvertent enterotomy during lysis of adhesions, or if a different surgical approach is chosen, the bowel will be adequately prepped so as to minimize contamination.

All patients receive 5000 units of heparin subcutaneously before induction of anesthesia. An arterial line is placed to assess potentially labile hemodynamics caused by a potential pneumothorax that can occur during the mediastinal dissection. The patient is positioned supine on the operating table with the arms abducted 45°.

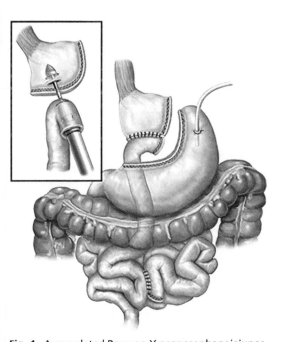

Fig. 1. A completed Roux-en-Y near esophagojejunostomy completed in a retrocolic and retrogastric fashion. The esophagojejunal anastomosis is performed with the use of an EEA stapler, shown in the inset. (*From* Awais O, Pennathur A, Luketich JD. Reoperative antireflux surgery. In: Luketich J, editor. Master techniques in surgery: esophageal surgery. Philadelphia: Wolters Kluwer Health; 2014. p. 93; with permission.)

A footboard is placed to support steep reverse-Trendelenburg positioning. If not previously done, an on-table endoscopy is performed to assess anatomic abnormalities and rule out any neoplastic lesions. Also, if present, the location and integrity of the previous wrap and the esophageal length can be evaluated. Care is taken to limit insufflation during endoscopy and to decompress the stomach on withdrawing of the scope. Iatrogenic distention of the stomach and small bowel can lead to injury during port placement as well as limiting visualization during dissection. The scope may also be left in the esophagus to aid in identification during dissection.

SURGICAL APPROACH

The surgeon works on the right with the assistant on the left. The first laparoscopic port is placed away from any previous incisions. In most instances, a blunt port using cut-down technique is place in the right upper quadrant. The abdomen is insufflated to 15 mm Hg and a 5-mm 30° camera is introduced into the abdomen. Once the peritoneal cavity is entered, inspection of the abdominal cavity is completed to ensure no injury was made on entrance. We then place additional ports under direct visualization. If needed, adhesiolysis is performed to allow our usual port placement used for laparoscopic antireflux surgery. Five ports are placed: a port in each midclavicular line just inferior to the costal margin, a port through each rectus muscle midway between the xiphoid and umbilicus approximately 4 cm away from each other, and a port in the right midaxillary line just inferior to the costal margin (**Fig. 3**). The right paramedian port is a 10-mm port to allow for instrumentation, all other ports are 5-mm ports. The patient is placed in a steep reverse-Trendelenburg position to displace the viscera from the diaphragm. A liver retractor (Lapro-Flex Triangular Retractor, Mediflex, Islandia, NY) is inserted through the right midaxillary port and the right crus is exposed. Usually in redo surgery, the left lateral segment of the liver is densely adherent and requires adhesiolysis before being able to place the liver retractor. Once all the appropriate ports are placed and adequate exposure is achieved, the surgery is commenced. The key principles of repairing recurrent PEHs are crural preservation, identification and preservation of vagal nerves, reduction of hernia sac and its contents, restoring normal anatomy, complete esophageal mobilization including mediastinal mobilization, mobilization of the gastroesophageal fat pad and assessment of whether esophageal length is adequate, appropriate crural closure, and

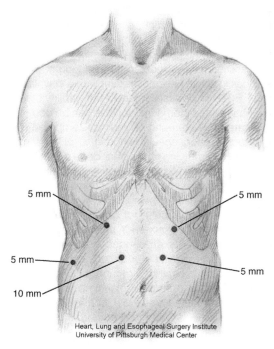

5 mm   5 mm
5 mm   5 mm
10 mm

Heart, Lung and Esophageal Surgery Institute
University of Pittsburgh Medical Center

Fig. 3. Laparoscopic port placement. (*From* Shah RD, Levy RM, Luketich JD. Minimally invasive Ivor Lewis esophagectomy. In: Luketich J, editor. Master techniques in surgery: esophageal surgery. Philadelphia: Wolters Kluwer Health; 2014. p. 275; with permission.)

performance of an antireflux procedure. The exact steps with additional description are detailed later.

SURGICAL PROCEDURE
Step One: Foregut Exposure

The most severe adhesions are encountered between the stomach, distal esophagus, and liver. In a hostile foregut, the caudate lobe of the liver is an important landmark in identifying the right crus. Once identified, a meticulous dissection is performed around the hiatus. In the cases in which mesh may have been used during the index operation, the adhesions tend to be more severe. If permanent mesh was used, it will need to be completely dissected and excised in order to expose the hiatus. During crural dissection, it is imperative to preserve the crural lining. The authors think this is pivotal when attempting to primarily close the hiatal defect. The hernia contents are reduced after adequate dissection allows reduction. It is critical to avoid perforation of the stomach and esophagus.

Step Two: Reduction of Hernia Sac/Mediastinal Dissection

The authors do not place traction on the stomach itself; we focus on dissecting and reducing the sac. This method reduces the stomach back into the abdomen. Once the hernia sac is identified, it is grasped inside the hiatus near the 12-o'clock position and everted. Then, using a hemostatic energy device, a window is made between the hernia sac and anterior peritoneal lining. An avascular, areolar plane should be encountered (**Fig. 4**). The plane is dissected into the mediastinum using a combination of blunt and sharp dissection. The dissection plane is along the posterior pericardium. The dissection should be carried up to the inferior pulmonary veins. The dissection is then performed circumferentially to the level of each pleural lining. In recurrent PEH, the hernia sac tends to be densely adhered to the pleural lining, and entry into the pleural space can easily be done during dissection. Entering the pleural space during mediastinal dissection is usually asymptomatic; however, in certain instances it can cause hypotension or increased airway pressures, which can be easily treated with placement of a chest tube or pigtail catheter.

During the mediastinal dissection, it is important to identify the esophagus and both vagi early to avoid any injury. If the endoscope was left in place at the start of operation, this may aid in identification. Every attempt should be made to identify the vagus nerves in order to preserve them during esophageal dissection. Once the dissection is performed circumferentially, complete right and left crural mobilization need to be accomplished if not already done. Once again, it is important to preserve

Careful preservation of crural muscle and peritoneal lining

Reduced hernia sac

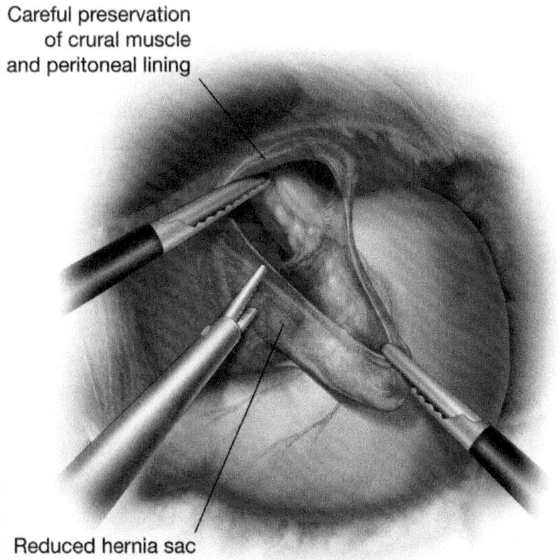

Fig. 4. Dissection of hernia sac. (*From* Nason KS, Luketich JD. Laparoscopic paraesophageal hernia repair. In: Luketich J, editor. Master techniques in surgery: esophageal surgery. Philadelphia: Wolters Kluwer Health; 2014. p. 127; with permission.)

the crural peritoneal lining because this preserves the integrity of the crura. Once the hiatus is completely mobilized, the mediastinal dissection is continued posteriorly between the esophagus and aorta. Note that, in reoperative cases, certain planes may be difficult. If at any point progress is not safe, we move to another area and reassess there.

Step Three: Restoration of Normal Anatomy

Once the hernia contents and sac are completely reduced, an attempt at restoring normal anatomy should be made. The authors think this is a critical step, and not only may it suggest the cause of failure, it allows a complete evaluation before deciding on the optimal repair. If a previous fundoplication was performed, we recommend a complete takedown of the previous repair, even if it appears to be intact and defining the gastroesophageal junction after dissection of the gastroesophageal fat pad. We generally start on the left limb of the wrap and sweep any fat or tissue centrally to avoid injury to the anterior vagus nerve. Removal of the fundoplication sutures can safely be done from the undersurface of the wrap. Once this is completed, the right limb can be freed in a similar manner. All adhesions to the stomach should be freed. If not done previously, the short gastric vessels need to be divided to completely mobilize the gastric cardia and fundus. Any retrogastric attachments should also be divided to allow the stomach to lay in the abdominal cavity in its normal orientation. Once the stomach is appropriately mobilized, the fundic tip should be able to be lifted easily and completely.

Step Four: Assessment of Intra-Abdominal Esophageal Length

Once normal anatomy is restored and the esophagus is fully mobilized in the mediastinum, and the gastroesophageal junction is defined after dissection of the gastroesophageal fat pad, the authors assess our intra-abdominal esophageal length. Ideally, 2.5 to 3 cm of tension-free intra-abdominal esophageal length should be established. Before assessing the length, we think it is critical, if not already done on a prior operation, to dissect off the anterior gastroesophageal fat pad to allow precise location of the gastroesophageal junction. The hernia sac that was reduced from the mediastinum can often be left in situ. However, if the sac is bulky and compromises the repair, excising and removing the hernia sac is recommended. It is important to remember that, when dissecting the fat pad and hernia sac, care must be taken to identify and preserve the vagus nerves, which tend to be incorporated into the fat pad and may be adherent to the hernia sac.

Step Five: Creation of Collis Gastroplasty (If Needed)

If adequate intra-abdominal esophageal length is not completed after complete mediastinal dissection, a Collis gastroplasty is performed. Our common approach is performing a wedge gastroplasty using linear staplers over a 52-Fr or 54-Fr bougie (**Fig. 5**).

Step Six: On-Table Endoscopy

Because of the complexity of reoperative esophageal surgery, the authors routinely repeat an on-table endoscopy after our mediastinal dissection is completed and normal anatomy is restored to evaluate any inadvertent esophageal or gastric perforations. If an injury is identified, it should be repaired before performing the fundoplication and hiatal closure. In rare instances, extensive damage to the gastroesophageal junction or fundus can alter surgical plans.

Step Seven: Creation of Fundoplication

Once the hernia sac and contents are completely reduced, there are several surgical options for how to proceed, as previously mentioned. Each approach should be individually tailored to each patient based on preoperative work-up and intraoperative findings. Because repair of a PEH disrupts the integrity of the lower esophageal antireflux barrier, the authors perform an antireflux procedure in most patients to prevent symptomatic reflux disease postoperatively. In our surgical practice, we most commonly proceed with a complete 360°-degree floppy fundoplication, and therefore our technique is described here.

When performing a complete wrap, we prefer a floppy, 2-stitch fundoplication on the esophagus over a 52-Fr to 56-Fr bougie or on the neoesophagus if a Collis gastroplasty was performed. Importantly, to minimize esophageal injury, the surgeon passes the bougie, with direct laparoscopic visualization. The fundoplication is created by passing the fundus left to right through the retroesophageal window with proper orientation using the line of the divided short gastric vessels. A shoeshine maneuver is performed to confirm proper orientation of the fundoplication. The 2-cm long fundoplication is secured using 2 simple interrupted 2-0 nonabsorbable sutures. Each stitch consists of full-thickness bites of stomach flanking a partial-thickness bite of esophagus to prevent wrap herniation (**Fig. 6**). Once the fundoplication is completed, the bougie is removed. For patients with severe dysmotility, a partial wrap (Dor or Toupet) may be considered.

Step Eight: Closure of Hiatal Defect

As previously mentioned, it is critical to preserve the crura with their peritoneal lining during the dissection, and this is an essential step in the successful repair of the hiatus. Whenever possible, our preferred approach to crural closure is a tension-free primary closure. The crura are approximated posterior to the esophagus with 2 or 3 interrupted sutures using a 0 nonabsorbable suture. Occasionally, an anterior stich is also required. In large defects, a tension-free repair can be challenging. Certain adjuncts that can be used to perform a primary crural repair include inducing a left-sided pneumothorax and reducing the intra-abdominal pressure during laparoscopy. If any degree of tension is noted while performing a crural repair, we induce a pneumothorax with close hemodynamic monitoring, and this allows the crura to be repaired without tension. Although some clinicians have used pledgets for the crural repair, with use of adjuncts, we have

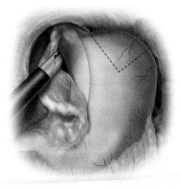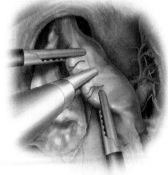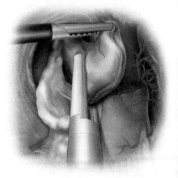

Fig. 5. Laparoscopic wedge Collis gastroplasty. (*From* Nason KS, Luketich JD. Laparoscopic paraesophageal hernia repair. In: Luketich J, editor. Master techniques in surgery: esophageal surgery. Philadelphia: Wolters Kluwer Health; 2014. p. 129; with permission.)

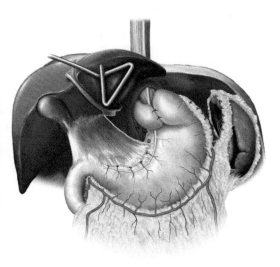

Fig. 6. Completed Nissen fundoplication. (*From* Awais O, Pennathur A, Luketich JD. Reoperative antireflux surgery. In: Luketich J, editor. Master techniques in surgery: esophageal surgery. Philadelphia: Wolters Kluwer Health; 2014. p. 92; with permission.)

not found this necessary.[11] At the completion of the repair, a grasper is introduced through the hiatus with an approximately 1 cm of space around the esophagus.

Despite the measures described earlier, if the crura cannot be reapproximated in a tension-free manner, a biologic mesh may be used to close the crural defect. Our current mesh of choice is Surgisis ES (Cook Surgical, Bloomington, IN). The mesh is secured to the diaphragm using 2-0 nonabsorbable suture or tacking device. Nonabsorbable mesh around the hiatus should be avoided at all costs because of the concern of delayed erosion into the esophagus.

Step Nine: Completion Endoscopy

The authors routinely repeat the endoscopy at the completion of the hiatal repair to ensure there is no compromise to the esophageal lumen. During endoscopy, areas to specifically evaluate the esophagus are at the level of the crural closure and the wrap. If the crura are closed too tightly it can prevent passage of endoluminal contents. Also, when large hiatal defects are present, the closure, whether primarily or with use of mesh, can cause angulation at the hiatal level, which can compromise passage of solids and/or liquids, leading to dysphagia. This situation can be assessed intraoperatively and should be corrected if noted.

Once we are satisfied with our repair, we place a 10-Fr Jackson-Pratt drain in the mediastinal space. This space can be large depending on

the size of the PEH and tends to fill with fluid in the immediate postoperative settings and occasionally is symptomatic. A nasogastric tube is also placed in close coordination with the surgeon and the anesthesiologist under laparoscopic visualization. This placement of a nasogastric tube is done with care, under direct visualization by the surgeon, and is particularly important to prevent esophageal injury. This tube is helpful in reducing postoperative retching or bloating, which can comprise the hiatal repair.

IMMEDIATE POSTOPERATIVE CARE

The care of the patients in the immediate postoperative period is similar for patients undergoing initial repair of PEH. All patients are usually extubated in the operating room and, after a short period in the recovery room, are transferred to a monitored bed. As mentioned previously, early vomiting or retching pose a significant risk to the integrity of the crural closure. Prophylaxis against nausea and vomiting is initiated before extubation and continued postoperatively with standing intravenous ondansetron 4 mg every 6 hours. Patients are started on patient-controlled analgesia until they can start oral intake. Early ambulation is encouraged. Nutritional and respiratory services are consulted to help with dietary education and pulmonary toilet, respectively.

The nasogastric tube is usually removed on postoperative day 2 and a barium contrast study is performed. If there is no leak and gastric emptying is acceptable, patients are started on a post-Nissen diet and transitioned to oral medications. The post-Nissen diet starts with noncarbonated clear liquids. The diet is not quantity based, but the patients are encouraged to start slowly and stop if they feel full. All medications should be crushed or given in liquid form. Patients are discharged home on oral ondansetron 4 mg every 8 hours and simethicone 80 mg every 6 hours. Patients are maintained on clear liquids for 3 days, followed by full liquids for 3 days, and then advanced to a soft diet until seen in follow-up. At the first outpatient follow-up, the diet restrictions are generally lifted with the exception of portion control.

After routine Nissen fundoplication without Collis gastroplasty, home proton pump inhibitors (PPIs) are discontinued. Patients undergoing Nissen fundoplication with Collis gastroplasty or gastropexy are discharged home on a daily PPI, which is eventually discontinued. The Jackson-Pratt drain that was placed in the mediastinal space is usually removed on postoperative day 3 before discharge.

REHABILITATION AND RECOVERY

Patients generally have their first postoperative appointment 2 weeks after discharge with a chest radiograph and are followed annually for a minimum of 5 years. Routine barium swallow is performed annually to assess overall function and anatomy. In the absence of symptom recurrence or anatomic abnormalities, patients follow up as needed after 5 years. Asymptomatic radiographic or endoscopic abnormalities are generally observed until symptoms develop. Surveillance EGD is not routinely performed except when symptoms develop.

In our experience, small recurrent hernias were associated with minimal symptoms and can be managed nonoperatively. The importance of routine surveillance barium swallows in the postoperative assessment is that they allow us to compare any changes over time. If a patient with a known recurrence develops worsening symptoms but has an unchanged barium esophagram, operative repair of the recurrence is unlikely to improve the patient's symptoms. In contrast, a patient with new or worsening symptoms along with findings of a new recurrence could be a candidate for reoperation.

The authors have instituted the use of validated measures (gastroesophageal reflux disease [GERD] health-related quality of life [HRQOL] and overall quality of life [Short Form 36]) to standardize symptom assessment. We found that having pathway-driven clinical follow-up, significant symptoms can be identified and appropriate therapy and/or intervention can be initiated. Symptoms in the postoperative phase include dysphagia, heartburn, and gas bloat. Most symptoms can be treated with diet and lifestyle modifications in addition to medical therapy. Some patients benefit from endoscopy and dilation, and, in extreme situations, a reoperation may be warranted.

RESULTS

The incidence of recurrent PEH can be up to 59%.[9] Recurrent PEHs present a challenging problem for surgeons. Although not completely clear, obesity[4] and an unrecognized short esophagus[12,13] are suggested as causes for an increased risk of recurrence. Wennergren and colleagues[14] also noted that Collis gastroplasty was required more frequently in redo PEH repair. Although some symptomatic patients with recurrent PEH can be treated nonoperatively, many patients who have significant moderate to severe symptoms require operative repair. Repair of recurrent PEH is warranted in these situations and can resolve related symptoms with good patient satisfaction.[9,14,15] In addition, all patients with moderate-sized or type IV recurrent PEH should be offered elective surgical repair because there is significant morbidity in urgent repairs.[4]

Before undergoing repair of recurrent PEH, patients require a comprehensive work-up. Work-up should include a detailed history and physical examination, review of prior operative notes, and appropriate diagnostic testing. Several different surgical options exist. However, each surgical approach needs to be tailored to each individual patient. The initial step to repair a recurrent PEH is similar to the initial repair, which is complete reduction of hernia sac and contents. Once this is completed, several options exist. Options for esophageal preservation include another fundoplication with or without a Collis gastroplasty, gastropexy, and a construction of a Roux-en-Y near esophagojejunostomy. The other option is an esophagectomy.

Redo hiatal surgery is complex. There are an associated increased number of complications with reoperative antireflux surgery,[16] and many patients require subsequent operations.[12] Further, the success rate of any antireflux surgery deceases in patients that had prior antireflux surgeries.[16] However, redo antireflux surgeries, although complex, can be done with a minimally invasive approach with good results.[12,17] Recurrent PEH can be performed safely as the initial PEH repair.[14]

Although there are several controversies in the repair of giant PEHs, generally, after complete reduction of hernia sac and contents, a fundoplication is performed. This procedure is normally done after the extensive sac dissection and reduction of the hernia because many of these hernias are type 3 hernias. As Pearson and colleagues[18] described, this is likely a result from progressive enlargement of a sliding component. Although first-time fundoplication provides symptomatic control in 90% of patients,[19] outcomes decline to ~80% or less after reoperative antireflux surgery.[20] In one of the largest series of redo antireflux surgery reported to date, at the University of Pittsburgh, we previously reported our experience in 275 patients who underwent redo antireflux surgery.[10] The most common pattern of failure of the initial operation was transmediastinal migration recurrent hernia in 177 patients (64%). Redo surgery included Nissen fundoplication in 200 patients (73%), Collis gastroplasty in 119 (43%), and partial fundoplication in 41 (15%). There was no perioperative mortality. The 2-year estimated probability of freedom from failure was 93%. The HRQOL scores, available for 186 patients, were excellent to satisfactory in 85.5% of patients.

Another esophageal preserving approach after hernia reduction is RNYNEJ (see **Fig. 1**). Our institution previously reported it as a good alternative for failed antireflux surgery in obese patients and those with esophageal dysmotility.[10] In another large series evaluating RNYNEJ for failed antireflux surgery, from the University of Pittsburgh, we reported the results of RNYNEJ for failed antireflux operations in 105 patients with BMI greater than 25. Most were obese (BMI>30; 82 patients [78%]); esophageal dysmotility was found in more than one-third of patients. Forty-eight (46%) patients had multiple antireflux operations before RNYNEJ, and 27 patients had undergone a previous Collis gastroplasty. There was no perioperative mortality. During follow-up, median BMI decreased from 35 to 27.6 ($P<.0001$), and the mean dysphagia score improved significantly ($P<.0001$). The median GERD-HRQOL score, assessed in a subset of patients, was classified as excellent. We concluded that RNYNEJ for persistent GERD after antireflux operations in appropriately selected patients can be performed safely with good results in experienced centers. RNYNEJ should be considered an important option for the treatment of intractable recurrent symptoms after antireflux operations, particularly in obese patients.

Not only did many patients have improvement in symptoms, they had associated benefits of weight loss and improvement in comorbid conditions. Some investigators have also reported that Roux-en-Y reconstruction is a better option for patients with a short esophagus compared with redo Collis gastroplasty.[15] The third option for esophageal preservation, which may be considered in highly selected patients with a minimal reflux history, is a gastropexy. Although this may put the patient at risk for reflux, there are certain situations, such as when the surgeon is concerned about the patient's stability or the viability of the stomach, in very elderly patients, in patients with significant multiple comorbidities, or in patients with a significant esophageal motility disorder, in which gastropexy may offer a better alternative. However, further analysis of outcomes after gastropexy needs to be done.

Although esophageal preservation is generally recommended, it is not always feasible. Factors that may favor esophagectomy include severe esophageal dysmotility, multiple prior operations, strictures, obstructive symptoms, and/or high-grade dysplasia/cancer.[21] Patients that have had prior hiatal surgery can have an esophagectomy with good results[22]; however, it is associated with higher morbidity, rates of anastomotic leaks, and reoperation.[21,23] It is also associated with a higher use of nongastric conduits.[22] Any patient with high suspicion of needing an esophagectomy should be evaluated for alternative conduits preoperatively. Overall, esophagectomy after prior hiatal hernia surgery is extremely challenging and carries a high morbidity. It should be performed by experienced esophageal surgeons at high-volume centers.

Another important aspect in initial or recurrent PEH repair is adequate closure of the hiatal defect. Although the authors are proponents of a primary tension-free closure, several investigators have advocated the use of mesh because it may decrease the rate of recurrence.[24–27] However, long-term studies in randomized trials did not show significant benefit for the mesh, and further studies are needed for definitive conclusions. One concern against the use of mesh is the risk of esophageal erosion. Therefore, we generally avoid the use of synthetic mesh if possible.

SUMMARY

Recurrent PEHs with significant associated symptoms can be very problematic and cause significant morbidity if left untreated. Surgical treatment of recurrent PEH can pose a great challenge. Several different surgical options are available and need to be considered on an individual basis. Before embarking on a recurrent repair, a thorough work-up needs to be completed, including a review of prior operative details and the use of imaging modalities. Although there are many approaches to repair, a minimally invasive approach can be performed by surgeons with extensive experience in minimally invasive esophageal surgery. Repair of recurrent PEH provides excellent patient satisfaction and symptoms resolution. Routine follow-up with surveillance imaging can assist in treatment of recurrent symptoms.

REFERENCES

1. Stylopoulos N, Gazelle GS, Rattner DW. Paraesophageal hernias: operation or observation? Ann Surg 2002;236(4):492–500 [discussion: 500–91].

2. Maziak DE, Todd TR, Pearson FG. Massive hiatus hernia: evaluation and surgical management. J Thorac Cardiovasc Surg 1998;115(1):53–60 [discussion: 61–2].

3. Diaz S, Brunt LM, Klingensmith ME, et al. Laparoscopic paraesophageal hernia repair, a challenging

operation: medium-term outcome of 116 patients. J Gastrointest Surg 2003;7(1):59–67.

4. Luketich JD, Nason KS, Christie NA, et al. Outcomes after a decade of laparoscopic giant paraesophageal hernia repair. J Thorac Cardiovasc Surg 2010; 139(2):395–404, 404.e1.

5. Nason KS, Luketich JD, Qureshi I, et al. Laparoscopic repair of giant paraesophageal hernia results in long-term patient satisfaction and a durable repair. J Gastrointest Surg 2008;12(12):2066–75 [discussion: 2075–7].

6. Pierre AF, Luketich JD, Fernando HC, et al. Results of laparoscopic repair of giant paraesophageal hernias: 200 consecutive patients. Ann Thorac Surg 2002;74(6):1909–15 [discussion: 1915–6].

7. Schauer PR, Ikramuddin S, McLaughlin RH, et al. Comparison of laparoscopic versus open repair of paraesophageal hernia. Am J Surg 1998;176(6): 659–65.

8. Mattar SG, Bowers SP, Galloway KD, et al. Long-term outcome of laparoscopic repair of paraesophageal hernia. Surg Endosc 2002;16(5): 745–9.

9. Kao AM, Otero J, Schlosser KA, et al. One more time: redo paraesophageal hernia repair results in safe, durable outcomes compared with primary repairs. Am Surg 2018;84(7):1138–45.

10. Awais O, Luketich JD, Reddy N, et al. Roux-en-Y near esophagojejunostomy for failed antireflux operations: outcomes in more than 100 patients. Ann Thorac Surg 2014;98(6):1905–11 [discussion: 1911–3].

11. Whitson BA, Hoang CD, Boettcher AK, et al. Wedge gastroplasty and reinforced crural repair: important components of laparoscopic giant or recurrent hiatal hernia repair. J Thorac Cardiovasc Surg 2006; 132(5):1196–202.e3.

12. Awais O, Luketich JD, Schuchert MJ, et al. Reoperative antireflux surgery for failed fundoplication: an analysis of outcomes in 275 patients. Ann Thorac Surg 2011;92(3):1083–9 [discussion: 1089–90].

13. Rathore MA, Andrabi SI, Bhatti MI, et al. Metaanalysis of recurrence after laparoscopic repair of paraesophageal hernia. JSLS 2007;11(4):456–60.

14. Wennergren J, Levy S, Bower C, et al. Revisional paraesophageal hernia repair outcomes compare favorably to initial operations. Surg Endosc 2016; 30(9):3854–60.

15. Juhasz A, Sundaram A, Hoshino M, et al. Outcomes of surgical management of symptomatic large recurrent hiatus hernia. Surg Endosc 2012; 26(6):1501–8.

16. Little AG, Ferguson MK, Skinner DB. Reoperation for failed antireflux operations. J Thorac Cardiovasc Surg 1986;91(4):511–7.

17. van Beek DB, Auyang ED, Soper NJ. A comprehensive review of laparoscopic redo fundoplication. Surg Endosc 2011;25(3):706–12.

18. Pearson FG, Cooper JD, Ilves R, et al. Massive hiatal hernia with incarceration: a report of 53 cases. Ann Thorac Surg 1983;35(1):45–51.

19. Pessaux P, Arnaud JP, Delattre JF, et al. Laparoscopic antireflux surgery: five-year results and beyond in 1340 patients. Arch Surg 2005;140(10): 946–51.

20. Furnee EJ, Draaisma WA, Broeders IA, et al. Surgical reintervention after failed antireflux surgery: a systematic review of the literature. J Gastrointest Surg 2009;13(8):1539–49.

21. Madenci AL, Reames BN, Chang AC, et al. Factors associated with rapid progression to esophagectomy for benign disease. J Am Coll Surg 2013; 217(5):889–95.

22. Chang AC, Lee JS, Sawicki KT, et al. Outcomes after esophagectomy in patients with prior antireflux or hiatal hernia surgery. Ann Thorac Surg 2010;89(4): 1015–21 [discussion: 1022–3].

23. Shen KR, Harrison-Phipps KM, Cassivi SD, et al. Esophagectomy after anti-reflux surgery. J Thorac Cardiovasc Surg 2010;139(4):969–75.

24. Champion JK, Rock D. Laparoscopic mesh cruroplasty for large paraesophageal hernias. Surg Endosc 2003;17(4):551–3.

25. Granderath FA, Carlson MA, Champion JK, et al. Prosthetic closure of the esophageal hiatus in large hiatal hernia repair and laparoscopic antireflux surgery. Surg Endosc 2006;20(3): 367–79.

26. Johnson JM, Carbonell AM, Carmody BJ, et al. Laparoscopic mesh hiatoplasty for paraesophageal hernias and fundoplications: a critical analysis of the available literature. Surg Endosc 2006;20(3): 362–6.

27. Oelschlager BK, Pellegrini CA, Hunter J, et al. Biologic prosthesis reduces recurrence after laparoscopic paraesophageal hernia repair: a multicenter, prospective, randomized trial. Ann Surg 2006; 244(4):481–90.

Transthoracic Paraesophageal Hernia Repair

James Matthew Reinersman, MD, Subrato J. Deb, MD, FCCP*

KEYWORDS

- Transthoracic • Paraesophageal hernia • Belsey Mark IV • Collis gastroplasty

KEY POINTS

- The transthoracic approach to paraesophageal hernias still has a place in the treatment of complicated foregut conditions.
- Foregut anatomy, as visualized through the chest, is unique and requires a complete appreciation of the structures present, particularly those within the abdomen that are not readily visualized.
- The esophagus is best isolated adjacent to the inferior pulmonary vein, which is often above the hernia and most readily controlled.
- If the gastroesophageal junction does not reduce easily into the abdominal cavity, an esophageal lengthening procedure should be completed.

INTRODUCTION

Paraesophageal hernia (PEH) is a recently described entity, only being recognized as significant in the early 20th century.[1] Although Henry Ingersoll Bowditch was the first to describe a PEH in his case series of postmortem findings in 1846, it was not until the initiation of radiography that PEH began to be diagnosed in living patients.[2,3] The first published work on hiatal hernia repair was by Angelo Soresi in 1919, which described a transabdominal approach to the hiatus, and this was then followed by Stuart Harrington publishing the experience at Mayo Clinic with 27 patients.[4,5] Transthoracic techniques were first published by Richard Sweet in 1950, detailing his technique, which included reducing the hernia, plication of the hernia sac, and crushing the phrenic nerve.[6] The success of Sweet led to others pursuing transthoracic repairs, which became the dominant method to approach PEH throughout most of the 20th century, with refinements by surgical luminaries such as Philip Allison and Norman Barrett.[7,8]

Ronald Belsey had the most significant impact upon the repair of paraesophageal hernias during the second half of the 20th century until the advent of the laparoscopy. The Belsey Mark IV operation was the result of many years of observation and iterations.[9] The procedure was called the Mark IV to delineate that multiple previous versions of the operation were unsatisfactory, which Belsey trialed from 1949 to 1955. Belsey only published the results of the Mark IV after meticulous minimum 5-year follow up in 1030 patients.[9] This article discusses the current status of transthoracic PEH repair. It focuses on: (1) the utility of this approach in the modern era of minimally invasive surgery, (2) relevant intrathoracic anatomy to this approach, (3) stepwise approach to the repair, (4) published outcomes of transthoracic repairs.

Disclosure Statement: The authors have nothing to disclose.
Division of Thoracic and Cardiovascular Surgery, Department of Surgery, University of Oklahoma Health Sciences Center, 800 Stanton L. Young Boulevard, Suite 9000, Oklahoma City, OK 73104, USA
* Corresponding author.
E-mail address: Subrato-Deb@ouhsc.edu

INDICATIONS FOR TRANSTHORACIC REPAIR

As with most surgical approaches, the utility of 1 technique over another depends on surgeon experience and comfort level. Approaches to the repair of PEH are no different. In the absence of randomized data, no 1 method can be proven to be superior to another. Despite the lack of consensus upon the indications for a transthoracic approach to the repair of paraesophageal hernias, some assumptions can be made. Several considerations for a transthoracic approach to PEH repair based upon the authors' experiences are listed:

1. History of multiple previous abdominal operations. Advanced abdominal adhesions, particularly from previous foregut procedures, can significantly affect safe visualization of the stomach and esophagus.
2. Morbid obesity. Obese patients not only have higher rates of recurrence, but excessive adipose tissue can significantly affect safe visualization of the foregut anatomy. This is particularly true during mobilization of the fundus and division of the gastrosplenic connections.
3. Shortened esophagus. In situations where extensive mobilization and/or an esophageal lengthening may be required, the transthoracic approach offers certain advantages. The surgeon has a clear delineation of anatomy for the safe dissection of the esophagus beyond the inferior pulmonary veins, regardless of left atrial size, which can limit laparoscopic esophageal mobilization. Secondly, the performance of an esophageal lengthening procedure (Collis gastroplasty), is facilitated via a transthoracic approach. A longer esophageal length can be gained by the transthoracic method in contrast to laparoscopic lengthening techniques.[10]
4. Giant hernias. When more than 50% of the stomach is herniated into the chest, the term giant PEH is applied. These hernias are typically type III and IV hernias with associated axial volvulus and obstructive symptoms. Although laparoscopic repair of such hernias is successful, traditional transthoracic correction offers direct visualization and safe dissection and reduction of the hernia.[11]
5. Perforation. Rupture of the stomach, or in some cases, the distal esophagus, secondary to a strangulated and obstructed PEH can pose significant challenges during surgery, because of disruption of the normal anatomic planes and inflammation. In this situation, a thoracotomy provides direct visualization for safer dissection, the ability to debride the mediastinum, and repair of the perforation with excellent visualization. Added benefits include the ability to extend the incision into a thoracolaparotomy for added exposure of the upper abdomen and the placement of a feeding tube.
6. Concomitant motility disorder. In situations where there is a functional disorder of the esophagus, a transthoracic approach facilitates the performance of a long esophageal myotomy and partial fundoplication. Furthermore, an epiphrenic diverticulectomy can be accomplished.

INTRATHORACIC FOREGUT ANATOMY

The following list describes relevant anatomy for the intrathoracic approach to PEH.

- The distal esophagus, including the gastroesophageal junction (GEJ) in the setting of a PEH, is a left thoracic organ and best approached via the left chest (Fig. 1).
- The esophagus can be mobilized all of the way up to the level of the aortic arch from the left chest for determination of esophageal length. Key landmarks for dissection include the junction of the left inferior pulmonary vein and posterolateral pericardium, where the inferior pulmonary vein enters and the esophagus (Fig. 2). This is a good point to find and isolate the esophagus, usually above or away from hernia at this point.
- Understanding the relation of the right and left crura as approached via the left chest is important for dissection and satisfactory repair. The left crus is usually easily identifiable during the dissection (Fig. 3). The right crus is generally the deepest structure in the dissection and can be difficult to define.
- Intraperitoneally deep to the right crus will be the caudate lobe of the liver and posterior to that the inferior vena cava.

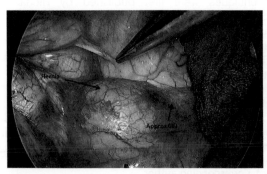

Fig. 1. Intrathoracic view of PEH. Arrows delineate intrathoracic stomach (hernia) and the approximate location of the GEJ.

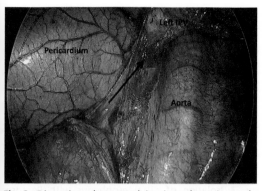

Fig. 2. Dissection plane overlying intrathoracic esophagus. The head is at the top of the picture. The confluence of the base of the left inferior pulmonary vein, posterolateral pericardium, and esophagus is highlighted with a black arrow and the ideal location to isolate the esophagus.

- Belsey's Artery is a collateral vessel between the ascending branch of the left gastric and the inferior phrenic artery (**Fig. 4**). This vessel, when present, runs through the superior portion of the gastrohepatic ligament. The key is to divide it from the chest securely, since it will retract into the abdomen and be inaccessible once divided.

HOW TO DO IT–TRANSTHORACIC REPAIR OF PARAESOPHAGEAL HERNIA
Planning/Preparation

Preoperative planning includes having a clear understanding of the anatomic and functional abnormalities prior to proceeding to the operating theater. This includes contrast imaging studies such as barium esophagram, computerized tomography of the thorax, and high- resolution manometry. High-resolution manometry may be difficult to obtain because of the distortion of the hiatus, and it is not always necessary.

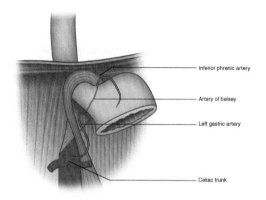

Fig. 4. Drawing depicting the location of the artery of Belsey.

Determination of fitness for surgery is critical to obtaining a good result. Physiologic parameters include evaluation of the cardiopulmonary system and estimation of the performance status. The authors' usual practice is to obtain pulmonary function testing in all patients undergoing thoracotomy.

Consideration for postoperative regional pain management, with epidural analgesia will aid in avoiding pulmonary complications following surgery.

Single-lung ventilation will facilitate exposure, although it is not mandatory. Lung isolation techniques include double lumen endotracheal intubation and bronchial blocker placement.

An orogastric tube is placed for gastric decompression. The patient is positioned in the right lateral decubitus position, and the left chest is prepared and draped widely, including the left upper quadrant of the abdomen.

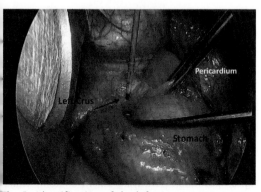

Fig. 3. Identification of the left crus.

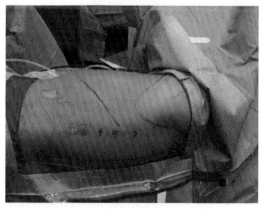

Fig. 5. External landmarks with the seventh interspace marked out for incision.

Incision and Exposure

Left muscle-sparing posterolateral thoracotomy, generally sixth or seventh intercostal space (top of seventh or eighth rib based on patient body habitus) is made (**Fig. 5**). The left lung is retracted medially and apically, exposing the posterior and inferior mediastinum. Next the inferior pulmonary ligament is taken down and the lung is packed in the upper thorax with a moist towel (**Fig. 6**). The junction of the esophagus, inferior pulmonary ligament, and pericardium is identified, and the mediastinal pleura over the esophagus is incised. The esophagus can be gently mobilized circumferentially, taking care to include the right and left vagus nerves, and then the esophagus can be encircled with a Penrose drain (**Figs. 7** and **8**).

Esophageal and Hernia Dissection

Dissection is extended superiorly to mobilize the esophagus for length, up to the level of the aortic arch, and inferiorly to the level of the hernia sac, staying right against the pericardium anteriorly to prevent injury to the vagus.

Next, start posterior dissection along sac–incision mediastinal pleura 1 cm anterior to

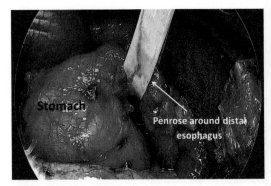

Fig. 7. Isolation of distal esophagus with Penrose drain.

descending thoracic aorta. Continue this dissection down once again until right pleura is encountered.

Follow the hernia sac then inferiorly until right crus is identified, taking care not to disrupt the fibers; grasp the right crus with a Babcock clamp. The lesser sac is then entered by going through the hernia sac between the crural fibers and the stomach. Once opened, the hernia sac is opened anteriorly and posteriorly.

Repair of Crural Defect

A Babcock clamp is placed on left crus, and the hernia sac is opened approximately 2 cm away from the crura so as to leave peritoneum on the crura for extra strength to the crural closure (**Fig. 9**).

Once the sac is opened, excise the sac from the crus and stomach; usually this can be accomplished bluntly with a Kitner dissector (**Fig. 10**). Stay 2 cm or more away from the vagus nerves

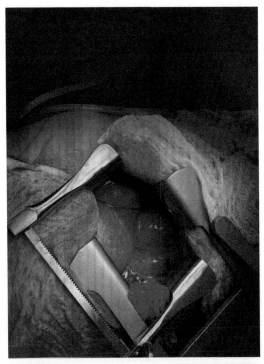

Fig. 6. Set up and exposure after thoracotomy; note heavy silk suture retracting the diaphragm caudally for improved exposure of the hiatus. The lung is packed in the upper thorax with a moist towel and is not seen.

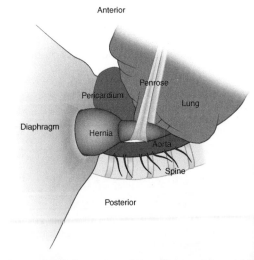

Fig. 8. Illustration portraying salient anatomy while mobilizing the esophagus.

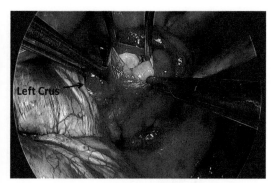

Fig. 9. Opening of hernia sac. Allis clamp on left crus of diaphragm, highlighted with black arrow.

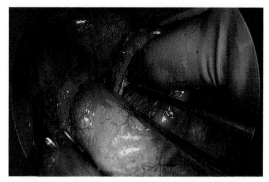

Fig. 11. View into lesser sac.

to avoid injury. Now that the sac is opened and removed, through the enlarged hiatus, the caudate lobe of the liver and lesser sac are visualized (**Fig. 11**). Gentle upward traction on the Penrose will identify any additional attachments to the peritoneum or phrenoesophageal ligament (**Fig. 12**). The GEJ fat pad is then excised. If the hernia is small, a few upper short gastric vessels may need to be divided; however, in large longstanding hernias, these are often elongated.

Following complete mobilization of the cardia and fundus, the GEJ is reduced back into the abdomen, and the crural repair is performed with either 0 or #1 Ethibond sutures (Ethicon Incorporated [Somerville, NJ], Ethibond Excel Polyester Suture) are placed from the right crus to the left, approximately 1 cm apart, and left untied (**Figs. 13** and **14**).

Belsey Mark IV Fundoplication

A Maloney dilator is passed through the esophagus at this point, usually 54 to 56 French.

The first layer of the Belsey is a series of 3 horizontal mattress sutures with the aim to create a 240° to 270° wrap. This is roughly the portion of the esophagus that lies between the right and left vagus nerves (**Fig. 15**).

First a seromuscular stitch on the stomach 2 cm away from the GEJ is placed, then through the esophageal muscle 2 cm above the GEJ, followed by the same parallel sutures in reverse (**Fig. 16**). Two more of the same sutures are placed in a 270° fashion, and then the sutures are tied down (**Fig. 17**).

The second layer is then constructed. A Belsey spoon or malleable is introduced into the abdomen to protect the abdominal viscera, and then the suture is passed through the diaphragm approximately 1 cm away from last crural repair suture. This suture is then continued through the seromuscular layer of the stomach 2 cm below the first row, and through the esophagus 2 cm above the first row and then brought back in reverse. An additional 2 sutures are placed in a similar manner to complete the 270° fundoplication (**Fig. 18**). The sutures are then tied after gently reducing the stomach back into the abdomen by grasping the esophagus with the right hand and pushing the stomach under the diaphragm with the thumb, ensuring no tissue is between the diaphragm and stomach.

The sutures are then tied, followed by tying the crural repair sutures (**Fig. 19**). The dilator is removed. The repair is tested by placing the tip of the index finger between the last crural suture

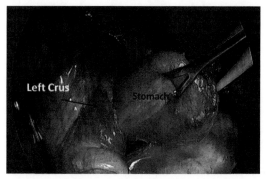

Fig. 12. Mobilization of the stomach through the hiatus.

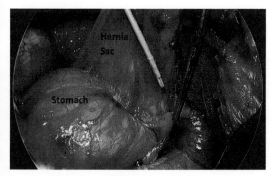

Fig. 10. Dissection of hernia sac.

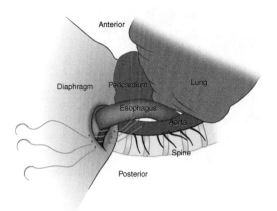

Fig. 13. Illustration detailing placement of posterior crural repair sutures.

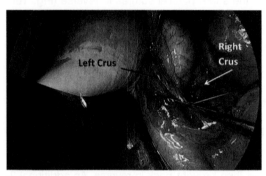

Fig. 14. Posterior crural repair; stomach temporarily reduced into the abdomen.

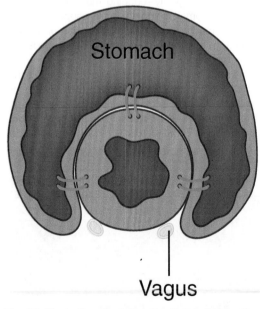

Fig. 15. Illustration depicting the Belsey fundoplication extending approximately 240° to 270° around the esophagus from left vagus to right vagus nerve.

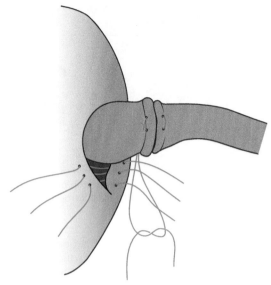

Fig. 16. Illustration showing the first layer of the Belsey fundoplication with untied crural closure sutures.

and the third Belsey fundoplication stitch. There should be enough room for the tip of the index finger with a bit of tension (**Fig. 20**).

Closure and Postoperative Management

Pleural drains are then placed; the left lung is re-inflated and the chest closed in the usual fashion. Routinely the authors do not utilize a postoperative nasogastric tube.

Patients are allowed clear liquids then are advanced to soft diet by the second or third day.

Monitoring for pulmonary complications requires vigilance. Incentive spirometry and ambulation are important.

The authors implement promotility therapy early following surgery, which is continued for 1 month. Venous thromboembolism prophylaxis is important, and the authors follow the Society of Thoracic Surgeons' recommendations on atrial fibrillation prophylaxis.

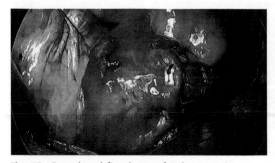

Fig. 17. Completed first layer of Belsey repair.

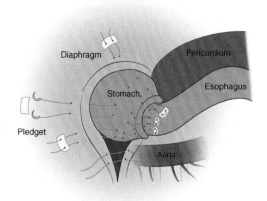

Fig. 18. Illustration depicting the second layer of the Belsey fundoplication and how it is constructed.

Patients are dismissed when they are taking adequate oral intake, and their pain is well controlled.

Transthoracic Nissen Fundoplication

A Nissen fundoplication can also be accomplished via the chest if the primary concern is postoperative reflux. This can be completed in a similar manner to the transabdominal approach, and often require short gastric vessel division to adequately mobilize the gastric fundus and eliminate tension on the wrap.

A transthoracic Nissen fundoplication can be performed if the patient has adequate motility and if reflux is a major consideration. The mobilization, hernia reduction and crural repair proceed in a similar fashion.

A 54 or 60 French Maloney dilator is placed, and the fundus is then brought around the distal esophagus, usually the distal 1.5 cm.

The wrap is then created in a 3-stitch technique with the middle stitch incorporating the

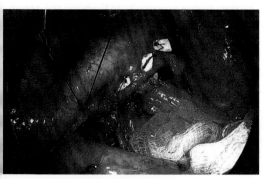

Fig. 19. View of completed Belsey repair, tying crural sutures. Note spacing of fundoplication sutures and crural repair sutures.

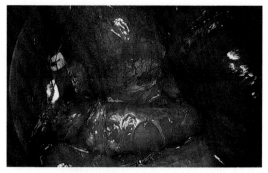

Fig. 20. Completed repair.

muscular layer of the esophagus. The fundoplication should be approximately 1.5 cm in length. The wrap is then reduced into the abdomen, crural sutures tied down, and the remainder is similar to what was described for the Belsey repair.

HOW TO DO IT–ESOPHAGEAL LENGTHENING

When employing the transthoracic repair for paraesophageal hernia, it is rare to be unable to mobilize the esophagus to have adequate intraabdominal length. However, when it is determined that there will be inadequate intra-abdominal esophagus, an esophageal lengthening procedure is employed. Options for transthoracic esophageal lengthening include Collis gastroplasty or a wedge gastroplasty.[12,13] The wedge gastroplasty was developed as an alternative to the Collis gastroplasty to be performed laparoscopically, because the Collis gastroplasty is easy to perform transthoracically but rather difficult laparoscopically, requiring multiple modifications, such as those highlighted by Luketich and colleagues, utilizing a combination of circular stapler and linear staplers.[14]

Collis Gastroplasty

The Collis gastroplasty is performed with the same 54 to 56 French dilator in place for the repair. The fundus and stomach should have already been sufficiently mobilized along with resection of the GEJ fat pad.

A linear endo-GIA stapler is introduced and placed parallel to the dilator across the gastric cardia along the fundus and fired. The staple line usually extends 5 cm from the GEJ inferiorly. This creates a gastric tube as the neo-esophagus to decrease tension (Fig. 21).

Wedge Gastroplasty

Alternatively, the wedge gastroplasty or fundectomy can be employed via the chest for

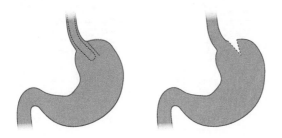

Fig. 21. Illustration of a Collis gastroplasty.

esophageal lengthening. Similar to the laparoscopic version, the fundus is elevated and straightened away from the cardia after placing a 54 to 56 French dilator.

A linear endo-GIA stapler is then utilized. Staple lines are made first along the greater curve. aiming toward the dilator and GEJ. Once the staple line is up to approximately the dilator, it is turned so that the staple line is parallel along the dilator toward the GEJ. The final result will be a wedge of fundus resected, creating a neo-esophagus to decrease tension (**Fig. 22**).

OUTCOMES OF TRANSTHORACIC REPAIR OF PARAESOPHAGEAL HERNIA

Since the writings of Skinner and Belsey in 1967,[9] contemporary results of the surgical outcomes of transthoracic surgery have been relatively sparse, partially because of the advent of laparoscopic techniques. In one of the largest experiences of transthoracic paraesophageal hernia repair, spanning 25 years at the University of Michigan, 240 patients with hernias underwent transthoracic surgery between 1977 and 2001.[15] Among this cohort, 92% were type III hernias and 8% were type IV. In this study, the operative approach was left thoracotomy via the sixth or seventh interspace. An esophageal lengthening procedure was performed in 96% of patients via Collis gastroplasty. Antireflux procedures included a Collis–

Nissen procedure in 96% of patients, Nissen fundoplication in 3% of patients, and a Belsey Mark IV fundoplication in 1% of patients. The results of surgery included death in 1.7% of patients and major complications in 8.5% of patients. Only 2 patients or less than 1% were presumed to have an esophageal perforation. On long-term follow-up, later recurrence of hernia was noted in 4 patients (<2%). Minor complications were noted in 13.8% of patients. This study was important in confirming that transthoracic approach can be done with low postoperative mortality and morbidity and compares favorably with transabdominal approaches.

Another large series from Toronto General Hospital evaluated the treatment of 94 patients with paraesophageal hernia between 1960 and 1990.[16] In this series, 50% of the patients had organo-axial volvulus. Of the 94 patients, 91 patients were treated with a transthoracic repair with fundoplication. A transthoracic Belsey Mark IV fundoplication was undertaken in all patients treated via the transthoracic route. An esophageal lengthening was performed in 80% of the patients with a Collis gastroplasty. Operative mortality was 2%. Significant complications occurred in 19% of patients. Four patients had a leak, with death resulting in 1 patient. The long-term results of follow-up in this study reveal 80% of patients with excellent results, 14% with good results, and 4% with fair results. Five patients had to undergo reoperation for a variety of reasons. Recurrent hernia rate was not discussed in this paper.

These 2 large experiences establish the transthoracic approach as a durable and safe approach with low mortality and acceptable morbidity and excellent functional outcomes. **Table 1** contrasts the largest laparoscopic experience to date out of the University of Pittsburgh, with some of the salient outcomes of the 2 largest transthoracic experiences discussed in this section.[11] It is clear that the outcomes are comparable with perhaps a slightly higher propensity to lengthen the esophagus in the transthoracic approaches.

TRANSTHORACIC VERSUS TRANSABDOMINAL APPROACHES

There are no randomized trials directly comparing open transthoracic versus open transabdominal or laparoscopic hiatal hernia repair. An analysis of outcomes using the National Surgical Quality Improvement Program (NSQIP) database between 2005 and 2011 evaluated 8186 patients who underwent PEH repair.[17] Utilizing multivariate analysis, the highest 30-day mortality was with an open transabdominal approach, with a 30-day

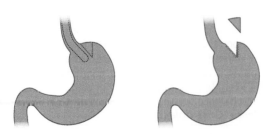

Fig. 22. Illustration of a wedge gastroplasty.

Table 1
Comparison of transthoracic to laparoscopic among the 3 largest series

Center (N)	Morbidity/ Mortality	Recurrence	Gastroplasty (%)	Fundoplication Type[a]	Outcome[b]
Michigan[15] (N = 240)	1.7%/8.5%	10%	96	Nissen	86%
Toronto[16] (N = 94)	2.0%/19%	2.1%	80	Belsey	94%
Pittsburgh[17] (N = 662)	1.7%/19%	15.7%	63	Nissen	89%

[a] Predominant fundoplication type in series.
[b] Outcomes include those with excellent and good functional result.

mortality of 2.6%. The transthoracic approach was 1.5%, and the laparoscopy approach had the lowest mortality of 0.5%. However, mean length of stay was statistically longer for open transabdominal and transthoracic approaches, compared with laparoscopy; an open abdominal procedure had a mean length of stay of 7.8 days, and transthoracic procedure had a mean length of stay of 6.5 days, compared with laparoscopy, which had a mean length of stay of 3.3 days.

A comparison between Belsey Mark IV and laparoscopic Nissen fundoplication in patients with large PEHs was undertaken by the Mayo Clinic.[18] In this single-center study, which encompassed a 10-year retrospective analysis evaluating 118 patients in each arm, the results revealed similar recurrence rates between patients who had a Belsey Mark IV and laparoscopic Nissen fundoplication, 8.4% versus 16.1%, P = .11. In this analysis, patients who underwent laparoscopic Nissen fundoplication had higher rates of reoperation at 9.3% versus 2.5%, and the leak rate was higher in patients who received a laparoscopic Nissen fundoplication compared with the transthoracic approach. These data emphasize that the tradeoff of lower morbidity with the laparoscopic approach has to be weighed against higher reoperation rates.

SUMMARY

The transthoracic approach to PEH has taken a back seat to minimally invasive approaches for valuable reasons; however, the well-trained esophageal surgeon will be quick to recognize that in select circumstances these may not be in the best interest of the patient or a successful operation. This article has discussed indications for a transthoracic approach, important anatomy, the steps of the procedure, and important outcomes associated with this repair.

REFERENCES

1. Allen MS. Belsey procedure- how I teach it. Ann Thorac Surg 2016;102:4–6.

2. Bowditch HI. A treatise on diaphragmatic hernia. Buffalo (NY): Jewett Thomas; 1853.

3. Stylopoulos N, Rattner DW. The history of hiatal hernia surgery: from Bowditch to laparoscopy. Ann Surg 2005;241:185–93.

4. Soresi AL. Diaphragmatic hernia: its unsuspected frequency: diagnosis and technique for radical cure. Ann Surg 1919;69:254–70.

5. Harrington SW. Diaphragmatic hernia. Arch Surg 1928;16:386–415.

6. Sweet RH. Diaphragmatic hernia. In: Sweet RH, editor. Thoracic surgery. Philadelphia: WB Saunders; 1950. p. 316–34.

7. Allison PR. Reflux esophagitis, sliding hiatal hernia and anatomy of repair. Surg Gynecol Obstet 1951; 92:419–431..

8. Barret NR. Hiatus hernia. Br J Surg 1954;42:231–43.

9. Skinner DB, Belsey RH. Surgical management of esophageal reflux and hiatus hernia: long-term results with 1,030 patients. J Thorac Cardiovasc Surg 1967;53:33–54.

10. DeMeester SR, Sillin LF, Lin HW, et al. Increasing esophageal length: a comparison of laparoscopic versus transthoracic esophageal mobilization with and without vagal trunk division in pigs. J Am Coll Surg 2003;197:558–64.

11. Luketich JD, Nason KS, Christie NA, et al. Outcomes after a decade of laparoscopic giant paraesophageal hernia repair. J Thorac Cardiovasc Surg 2010; 139:395–404.

12. Pearson FG. The collis-belsey procedure. Op Tech Card Thorac Surg 1997;2:52–60.

13. Whitson BA, Hoang CD, Boettcher AD, et al. Wedge gastroplasty and reinforced crural repair: important components of laparoscopic giant or recurrent hiatal hernia repair. J Thorac Cardiovasc Surg 2006;132: 1196–202.

14. Luketich JD, Raja S, Fernando HC, et al. Laparoscopic repair of giant paraesophageal hernia: 100 consecutive cases. Ann Surg 2000;232: 608–18.

15. Patel HJ, Tan BB, Yee J, et al. A 25 year experience with open primary transthoracic repair of paraesophageal hiatial hernia. J Thorac Cardiovasc Surg 2004;127:843–9.

16. Maziak DE, Todd TRJ, Pearson FG. Massive hiatus hernia: Evaluation and surgical management. J Thorac Cardiovasc Surg 1998;115: 53–62.

17. Mungo B, Molena D, Stem M, et al. Thirty-day outcomes of paraesophageal hernia repair using the NSQIP database: should laparoscopy be the standard of care? J Am Coll Surg 2014;219: 229–36.

18. Laan DV, Agzarina J, Harmsen WS, et al. A comparison between Belsey Mark IV and laparoscopic Nissen fundoplication in patients with large paraesophageal hernia. J Thorac Cardiovasc Surg 2018;156:418–28.

Anesthetic Management for Paraesophageal Hernia Repair

Tatiana Kazakova, MD[a], Bradley Hammond, DO[b], Chad Talarek, MD[b],
Ashish C. Sinha, MD, PhD, MBA[b], Neil W. Brister, PhD, MD[c],*

KEYWORDS

- Paraesophageal hernia • Carbon dioxide insufflation-pathophysiology • Aspiration risk
- Anesthetic management • Intraoperative complications • Pain control

KEY POINTS

- Preoperative symptoms related to the paraesophageal hernia may overlap with those of the cardio-pulmonary system in elderly patients.
- Symptoms need to be elicited to assess their increased aspiration risk and the need for a rapid sequence intubation with cricoid pressure.
- After induction of anesthesia, there are a variety of issues affecting the care of patients including ventilation, lung isolation, gastric tube placement, bougie insertion, fluid management, and degree of muscle relaxation.
- Intraoperative complications related to the surgical suite and techniques include hypotension, hypoxemia, pneumothorax, and subcutaneous emphysema.
- Multimodal pain control is discussed.

CLINICAL PRESENTATION/EPIDEMIOLOGY

A paraesophageal hernia (PEH) is defined as the herniation of the stomach and rarely additional viscera through the hiatus of the diaphragm, into the mediastinum. The herniation results from widening of the space between the diaphragmatic crura, allowing for protrusion of the abdominal contents into the chest cavity. PEHs are classified into four types based on location of the gastro-esophageal junction and the abdominal organ involved in the herniation.[1]

Patients with PEH present with a wide variety of symptoms, often related to the severity and acuity of herniation. Although PEH may present acutely, most cases are chronic and typically present in the sixth to seventh decade of life.

A sliding hernia, type I, accounts for approximately 90% of all hiatal hernias and are often asymptomatic.[2] However, gastroesophageal reflux disease may be present, leading to heartburn, regurgitation, cough, or chest pain. Long-term gastro-esophageal reflux disease can lead to erosive esophagitis, Barrett esophagus, and esophageal cancer. Larger defects, types II to IV, are more likely to present with progressive intolerance to food, and nausea, vomiting, and regurgitation. Herniation of abdominal contents may cause cardiopulmonary symptoms, such as chest pain, shortness of breath, arrhythmia, or exacerbation of an underlying chronic

Disclosure Statement: All authors have nothing to disclose.
[a] Department of Family Medicine, Jefferson Health NE, 10800 Knights Road, Philadelphia, PA 19114, USA;
[b] Department of Anesthesiology, Temple University Hospital, 3401 North Broad Street, B300 Outpatient Building Floor, Philadelphia, PA 19140, USA; [c] Department of Anesthesiology, Temple University Hospital, 3401 North Broad Street, B307 Outpatient Building Floor, Philadelphia, PA 19140, USA
* Corresponding author. 3401 North Broad Street B300 Outpatient Building, Philadelphia, PA 19140.
E-mail address: Neil.Brister@temple.edu

lung condition, such as chronic obstructive pulmonary disease or asthma.[3] Gastrointestinal bleeding and anemia may be present: iron deficiency results from chronic blood loss caused by a partially incarcerated and congested or ischemic stomach.[4] PEH can present acutely as a result of gastric obstruction, volvulus, incarceration, and strangulation. Acute presentations, up to 7% of patients per year, often require emergent surgical intervention.[5,6]

SURGICAL REPAIR

Over the past two decades, laparoscopic and robotic transabdominal repair have gained prevalence, because of a decrease in perioperative complications and length of stay.[7] In select cases, such as prior abdominal surgeries or recurrent PEH, a transthoracic approach, usually by open thoracotomy to the hiatus, may be preferred. Such procedures require management of standard thoracic anesthesia ventilatory challenges, including lung isolation.[7,8]

PREOPERATIVE EVALUATION OF PATIENTS

Preoperative evaluation includes a comprehensive history focusing on previous anesthetic experience, adverse events, difficult intubation, aspiration risk, elicitation of cardiopulmonary symptoms, and physical examination. Medical optimization should also focus on an extensive review of the patient's cardiopulmonary reserve and nutritional state. Ideally, medical optimization is achieved before elective surgery.

ASSESSMENT OF PULMONARY RISK

Baseline pulmonary status is particularly relevant in the preoperative assessment. Evidence of chronic aspiration should be sought, including chronic cough, pneumonia, bronchitis, or reactive airway disease. Major perioperative respiratory complications, such as atelectasis, aspiration, pneumonia, and respiratory failure, are a significant cause of morbidity and mortality, because surgery of the upper abdomen and thorax in itself may also be associated with pulmonary complications.[9] In addition, preoperative cessation of smoking should be strongly encouraged.[10]

ASSESSMENT OF ASPIRATION RISK

The PEH population is at high risk of aspiration during the induction of general anesthesia.[11] Accordingly, patients should be made aware of potential adverse outcomes associated with aspiration. It is imperative that preoperative fasting guidelines are followed. Preoperative antacids and gastrointestinal stimulants (ie, metoclopramide) should be continued on the day of surgery.[12] Vigilance should be exercised in ensuring that the patient is not having an acute exacerbation of symptoms, which would further increase their aspiration risk. Many patients are placed on a liquid diet for up to 72 hours before the procedure to help facilitate optimal surgical conditions and decrease aspiration risk.

ASSESSMENT OF CARDIOVASCULAR RISK

Cardiovascular complications are a potential cause of perioperative morbidity and mortality. Recent Guidelines for Perioperative Cardiovascular Evaluation for Noncardiac Surgery provide a framework for cardiac risk stratification.[13] Elderly patients with PEH are at elevated risk for adverse cardiac events, particularly atrial arrhythmias. There may be overlap in symptoms with regard to PEH and underlying cardiac disease. The origin of the symptoms must be clarified before elective surgery. Echocardiogram may be indicated for evaluation of valvular heart disease and congestive heart failure.

ANTICOAGULATION MANAGEMENT

Thoracic epidural analgesia is frequently used for pain control in open PEH repair. However, antiplatelet and anticoagulation medications may dictate suitability for thoracic epidural analgesia. According to guidelines published by the American Society of Anesthesia and Pain Medicine, P2Y12 inhibitors should be stopped for 7 days before moderate- to high-risk procedures, and may be restarted 12 hours post-procedure.[14] Warfarin should be stopped for 5 days and the international normalized ratio normalized before the procedure. It is restarted the following day. Intravenous heparin should be stopped for 6 hours before the procedure and is restarted 24 hours following the procedure. For subcutaneous twice a day or three times a day heparin dosing, the procedure is performed 6 hours after discontinuation and heparin dosing is restarted 6 to 8 hours after the procedure. Low-molecular-weight heparin in prophylactic dosing requires a 12-hour interval between discontinuation and the procedure, whereas a therapeutic dose requires a window of 24 hours. The low-molecular-weight heparin is restarted 12 hours following the procedure. Patients at high risk for thromboembolism should be bridged perioperatively, typically with low-molecular-weight heparin or unfractionated heparin.[15] In patients, receiving antiplatelet therapy after coronary stenting, delaying surgical intervention for at least 6 months for drug-eluding stents and 1 month for bare metal stents is recommended.[16]

ANESTHESIA MANAGEMENT

Intraoperative anesthetic management is divided into monitoring, induction and airway management, maintenance of anesthesia, and emergence.

MONITORING

Standard intraoperative monitoring includes: electrocardiogram, noninvasive blood pressure, pulse oximetry, continuous waveform capnography, and temperature. During laparoscopic procedures, fluid status is influenced by the effects of anesthetic agents, pneumoperitoneum, increased intra-abdominal pressure, and reverse Trendelenburg position.[17,18] Urine output monitoring is limited in guiding intraoperative fluid therapy. When significant comorbid conditions dictate, an arterial line may be appropriate for more fastidious blood pressure monitoring and blood gas sampling. In addition, noninvasive arterial monitors (ClearSight System [Edwards Lifesciences Corporation, Irvine, CA]) may provide further cardiac parameters in higher risk patients.[19,20] Changing levels of end-tidal carbon dioxide (P_{ETCO2}) can reflect increased absorption of insufflated CO_2 or portend possible inadequate ventilation, gas embolus, or pneumothorax. Patients with significant pulmonary disease and retention of CO_2 may benefits from monitoring arterial blood gases.

INDUCTION AND AIRWAY MANAGEMENT

Induction of anesthesia is accomplished by use of benzodiazepines, opioids, and hypnotic agents (propofol, etomidate, or ketamine). Neuromuscular blocking agents (NMBA) achieve muscle relaxation, facilitate endotracheal intubation, and may decrease insufflation pressure while maintaining pneumoperitoneum. Benzodiazepines provide anxiolysis and amnesia but may produce delayed emergence or disorientation postoperatively. Opioids provide analgesia and act to blunt sympathetic response to noxious stimuli. Adverse effects related to opioid use include respiratory depression, nausea and vomiting, and drowsiness. As such, dosing should be limited to that required to achieve therapeutic effect.[21–23] Hypnotic agents induce unconsciousness.

Preoperative airway examination aids in establishing a plan for the induction of anesthesia and intubation. Because of the high risk of aspiration, a rapid sequence intubation is frequently used. The patient is preoxygenated, and then administered a hypnotic agent, and rapid-acting muscle relaxant, in rapid succession with the goal of securing the airway as quickly as possible. Cricoid pressure (**Fig. 1**), although controversial, is often used in conjunction with rapid sequence intubation to compress the esophagus and prevent passive regurgitation of gastric contents. Cricoid pressure has been known to cause lateral displacement of the esophagus, decrease lower esophageal sphincter tone, and compress the airway, which can complicate intubation or even cause trauma.[24–26] The reverse Trendelenburg position during induction improves pulmonary mechanics and reduces the reflux of gastric contents, especially in obese patients.[27,28] Rapid intubation with cricoid pressure continues to be considered the safest way to secure the airway and reduce risk of aspiration.[29]

LUNG ISOLATION

Either a planned transthoracic surgical approach or intraoperative conversion to thoracotomy may require lung isolation. A double-lumen endotracheal tube or bronchial blockers is used to achieve lung isolation or one-lung ventilation. Double-lumen endotracheal tubes allow airway suctioning, lower incidence of intraoperative displacement, and may produce more rapid lung collapse.

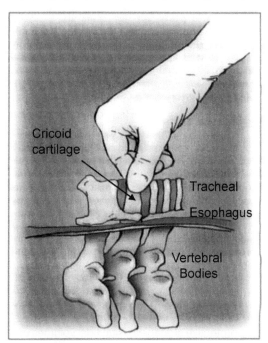

Fig. 1. Cricoid pressure. (*Modified from* Koziol CA, Cuddeford JD, Moos DD. Assessing the force generated with application of cricoid pressure. AORN J. 2000;72(6):1019; with permission.)

However, their larger profile makes them less amendable to placement in the difficult airway and more likely to induce airway trauma. Bronchial blockers are placed readily through an existing single-lumen endotracheal with fiberoptic guidance and are easily removed without tube exchange following the procedure. They are opportune in situations of anticipated difficult airway. However, the shorter length of the right main bronchus may result in inadequate isolation of the right upper lobe when right lung isolation is required. Lung isolation for thoracotomy is achieved with comparable quality of lung deflation regardless of whether double-lumen endotracheal tubes or bronchial blockers are used. Regardless of lung isolation method, fiberoptic bronchoscopy and knowledge of tracheal anatomy are required in their placement.[30,31]

ANESTHETIC MAINTENANCE

The anesthetic maintenance phase is accomplished by intravenous and inhalation agents, or a combination of both, providing amnesia and analgesia during the induced state of unconsciousness. Inhalation agents provide fine titratable control over anesthetic depth, although high doses of these potent agents can lead to postoperative nausea and vomiting, cardiac depression, hypotension, and ventilation–perfusion mismatch.[32,33] Inhibition of hypoxic pulmonary vasoconstriction may affect oxygenation during lung isolation. Inhalation agents typically provide more rapid emergence from anesthesia in comparison with intravenous anesthetics.[34] Total intravenous anesthesia is an alternative to volatile anesthetics.

In addition to facilitating intubation and mechanical ventilation, NMBAs optimize surgical exposure. "Deep" neuromuscular blockade may decrease insufflation pressure while maintaining pneumoperitoneum and optimize surgical exposure. Unexpected patient movement during laparoscopic surgery can result in injury.[35] This is especially important in robotic surgery while the robot is docked to metal ports that are inserted inside the patient. Reversal of NMBAs is typically achieved with neostigmine/glycopyrrolate or sugammadex, which is superior to neostigmine as a reversal agent.[36]

MECHANICAL VENTILATION

Lung-protective strategies using tidal volumes of 6 to 8 mL/kg of ideal body weight, and application of positive end-expiratory pressure of 5 to 10 cm H_2O should be used.[37] Reverse Trendelenburg position during the surgical procedure may improve ventilation parameters. Elevated arterial CO_2 may occur because of absorption of insufflated CO_2, requiring moderate hyperventilation. Mild permissive hypercapnia is deemed acceptable and is generally well tolerated. Recruitment maneuvers can mitigate the negative effects of pneumoperitoneum on pulmonary mechanics.[38]

FLUID MANAGEMENT

Preoperative fluid deficits may be substantial, because of preoperative fasts superimposed on baseline diminished oral intake.[4] Relative hypovolemia is common in a malnourished population. Minimally invasive repairs generally have low fluid requirements, because insensible losses are generally decreased in laparoscopic repairs. Both extremes (hypovolemia and hypervolemia) are associated with increased morbidity, including cardiorespiratory failure, kidney injury, compromised wound healing and staple line integrity, and abdominal compartment syndrome.[39] For major elective surgical procedures, goal-directed fluid management is recommended.[40,41]

INTRAOPERATIVE GASTRIC DRAINAGE

Placement of a gastric tube, via nasal or oral route, is commonly performed after intubation. However, in most foregut procedures, surgeons perform preoperative endoscopy for assessment of anatomy. Furthermore, because of anatomic variations created by PEH, placement of a gastric tube may be unsafe before dissection and mobilization of the stomach.[42] Discussion with the surgeon before placement of a gastric drain is vital.

PLACEMENT OF ESOPHAGEAL BOUGIES

To diminish the incidence of long-term dysphagia, a bougie may be used to support proper calibration of the fundoplication, preventing creation of an excessively tight wrap.[43,44] Additionally, if the surgeon determines that an esophageal lengthening procedure is required, this may also require intraoperative placement of an esophageal bougie to ensure adequate diameter of the neoesophagus.

Bougies are long, tapered tubes, available in various sizes and traditionally used for stricture dilations. The Maloney bougie is commonly used in PEH repair.[45] The Savary dilator is similar with the added advantage that it can be passed over a wire. This wire is passed through a gastroscope, greatly improving the ease and safety of the insertion.

Pre-existing esophageal pathology, excessive force or incorrect insertion technique, and improper traction on the stomach and esophagus during passage all create an increased risk for perforation.[43] Training of anesthesia personnel in bougie passage technique helps to reduce risk of perforation. A liberal amount of lubricant should be used. The operator may insert the index finger into the patient's mouth to guide the bougie through the hypopharynx and into the esophagus. Gentle pressure should be applied, carefully alternating clockwise and counterclockwise motion. If any atypical resistance is encountered, the surgeon should be notified.[46] Typically, the surgeon controls depth advancement of the bougie indirectly via laparoscopic view.

INTRAOPERATIVE COMPLICATIONS

Pneumoperitoneum and increased intra-abdominal pressure, and complex anatomy and proximity to vital structures predispose the patient to a variety of intraoperative complications.

Hypotension may result secondary to mechanical effects of pneumoperitoneum, whereby compression of the interior vena cava reduces venous return, decreasing cardiac preload and cardiac output. Positive pressure ventilation, reverse Trendelenburg positioning, induction and inhalation anesthetic agents, and preoperative fasting also contribute to decreased venous return. Minimizing intra-abdominal pressure (≤ 12 mm Hg for insufflation pressure), adequate fluid resuscitation, reduction in the degree of reverse Trendelenburg positioning, and low-dose vasopressors may help to maintain appropriate blood pressure.[47]

Hypoxemia during laparoscopic procedures is uncommon. It might be related to development of intraoperative pneumothorax or, in the case of single-lung ventilation, because of ventilation–perfusion mismatch. Thorough and prompt investigation of the underlying cause is paramount to appropriately address the condition. In the case of one-lung ventilation, inflating the previously isolated lung improves hypoxemia.

Subcutaneous emphysema during laparoscopic procedures results from insufflated CO_2 passing beyond the diaphragm to the mediastinum, where it goes on to track in the subcutaneous tissue planes. Typically, a pronounced increase in P_{ETCO2} and $Paco_2$ occurs, with subcutaneous emphysema of the head, neck, and thorax being noted. Because of high solubility of CO_2 in the blood, subcutaneous emphysema is generally a benign, self-limited condition. However, ventilation should be increased, pneumothorax ruled out, and compressive upper airway obstruction also ruled out following the procedure.[48]

Pneumothorax in the setting of esophageal surgery has several potential etiologies. Diaphragmatic defects may create pleura-peritoneal communication, whereas insufflation of the abdomen generates a pressure gradient favoring movement of gas into the mediastinum. In addition, manipulation of the tissue space surrounding the esophageal hiatus during dissection may allow insufflated gas to track along weak tissue planes superiorly and into the mediastinum, particularly affecting the left pleura. Finally, direct disruption of the pleura can create pneumothorax.[48] An abrupt increase in P_{ETCO2} is typically the initial manifestation of pneumothorax. Decreased lung compliance, elevated peak airway pressure, and decreased oxygen saturation as measured by pulse oximetry also occur. However, the most compelling evidence for pneumothorax is direct visualization of the entry point into the left pleural space.[49] Because of ease of absorption, intraoperative CO_2 pneumothorax is generally tolerated without the need for tube thoracostomy.

Hemopericardium/tamponade is a rare, but potentially fatal complication caused by transdiaphragmatic cardiac injury.[50–52] Suspicion should be triggered by development of hemodynamic instability. Although transesophageal echocardiography (TEE) readily identifies the pericardial effusion, an unstable patient exhibiting tamponade physiology may not tolerate delays for TEE. The surgical team should be alerted immediately. A transdiaphragmatic laparoscopic pericardial window or pericardiocentesis establishes the diagnosis and relieves the tamponade in preparation for a more definitive procedure.[53,54]

Gas embolism causing hemodynamically significant CO_2 embolism is rare because of the high solubility of CO_2 in the blood. However, macro emboli creating "air lock" can produce an abrupt decrease in P_{ETCO2}, increase in $Paco_2$, "millwheel" murmur, decrease in cardiac output and systemic blood pressure, and cardiovascular collapse.[48] Etiologies of CO_2 emboli include inadvertent placement of the gas insufflation needle into a blood vessel during insufflation, or more likely, venous laceration during laparoscopic dissection. The adverse effects of CO_2 embolism depend on volume of gas and rate of injection and the pathophysiologic effects result from accumulation of gas in the pulmonary circulation.[55] TEE is the gold standard for detection of a gas embolus. Treatment should include left lateral positioning with the head down, cessation of gas insufflation, release of pneumoperitoneum, and possibly aspiration of air from a central venous catheter. In the case of hemodynamic collapse, cardiopulmonary bypass may be required.[48]

Intraoperatively pulmonary embolism (PE) is an infrequent event, but potentially, a significant and fatal complication. Risk factors include obesity, oral contraceptive use, hormone-replacement therapy, prolonged immobilization, and previous PE. Peritoneal insufflation increases intra-abdominal pressure and when combined with reverse Trendelenburg position, contributes to lower extremity venous stasis and thrombosis. Classic symptoms are often concealed in patients under general anesthesia. An abrupt decline in P_{ETCO2} with a rise in $Paco_2$, or hemodynamic instability, may be the only early sign of intraoperative PE. TEE is performed quickly and with reasonable accuracy in patients with clinical suspicion of PE and evidence of right ventricle strain.[56] In the absence of visualization of thrombus in the pulmonary vasculature, right ventricle dilation and hypokinesis, septal shift, and tricuspid regurgitation are TEE findings consistent with PE.[57] Supportive therapy includes vasopressors, to improve right ventricle coronary perfusion pressure and contractility. Anticoagulant and thrombolytic therapies are controversial, because surgical patients are at increased risk of bleeding. Surgical embolectomy may be the only option for the hemodynamically unstable surgical patient.[57]

EMERGENCE AND POSTOPERATIVE CARE

The major goal of postoperative anesthetic care is a smooth transition from general anesthesia to the awake state of the patient. Emergence from anesthesia is a risky period.

PAIN CONTROL

Intraoperative opioids are commonly used as part of the anesthetic management and provide postoperative pain control. However, adverse effects include respiratory depression, nausea, vomiting, constipation, and drowsiness. Dosing should be aimed to achieve the optimal therapeutic effect.[21,23] Postoperative pain following minimally invasive repair is generally of less intensity and shorter duration. Some patients may experience predominantly visceral or referred pain. Specifically, shoulder pain can result from irritation of the phrenic nerve, secondary to diaphragmatic distention, residual subdiaphragmatic CO_2, and closure of the hiatus.[58,59] Multimodal analgesia has been shown to provide optimal pain control. Parenteral glucocorticoids (eg, dexamethasone) are used because of ability to reduce postoperative pain. Local infiltration of laparoscopic port sites provides short-term pain control. Continuous local anesthetic infusion may prolong duration of analgesia, especially with larger incisions. The transversus abdominis plane block may be beneficial.[60,61] Epidural analgesia provides excellent pain relief with improved outcomes after open abdominal surgery; however, potential risks of adverse effects, such as hemodynamic instability, postural hypotension, urinary retention, and delayed ambulation, make it less desirable with minimally invasive surgery.[60] Liposomal bupivacaine was shown to confer excellent pain control in many postoperative patients.[62]

Oral opioids are used for low to moderate postoperative pain if relief is inadequate with use of nonsteroidal anti-inflammatory drugs, nonopioid analgesics, or cyclooxygenase type 2–specific inhibitors when appropriate.[63,64] Implementation of enhanced recovery protocols has improved outcomes with faster recovery and decreased complications.[60,65,66]

REFERENCES

1. Oleynikov D, Jolley JM. Paraesophageal hernia. Surg Clin North Am 2015;95(3):555–65.
2. Kahrilas PJ, Lin S, Chen J, et al. The effect of hiatus hernia on gastro-oesophageal junction pressure. Gut 1999;44(4):476–82.
3. Gnanenthiran SR, Naoum C, Kilborn MJ, et al. Posterior cardiac compression from a large hiatal hernia: a novel cause of ventricular tachycardia. HeartRhythm Case Rep 2018;4(8):362–6.
4. Clark LN, Helm MC, Higgins R, et al. The impact of preoperative anemia and malnutrition on outcomes in paraesophageal hernia repair. Surg Endosc 2018;32(11):4666–72.
5. Hoff R, Qazi B. Strangulated paraesophageal hiatal hernia. J Am Osteopath Assoc 2018;118(3):207.
6. Sihvo EI, Salo JA, Rasanen JV, et al. Fatal complications of adult paraesophageal hernia: a population-based study. J Thorac Cardiovasc Surg 2009; 137(2):419–24.
7. Vasudevan V, Reusche R, Nelson E, et al. Robotic paraesophageal hernia repair: a single-center experience and systematic review. J Robot Surg 2018; 12(1):81–6.
8. El Lakis MA, Kaplan SJ, Hubka M, et al. The importance of age on short-term outcomes associated with repair of giant paraesophageal hernias. Ann Thorac Surg 2017;103(6):1700–9.
9. Canet J, Mazo V. Postoperative pulmonary complications. Minerva Anestesiol 2010;76(2):138–43.
10. Kulaylat AS, Hollenbeak CS, Soybel DI. Cost-utility analysis of smoking cessation to prevent operative complications following elective abdominal colon surgery. Am J Surg 2018;216(6):1082–9.
11. de Souza DG, Gaughen CL. Aspiration risk after esophagectomy. Anesth Analg 2009;109(4):1352.

12. Practice guidelines for preoperative fasting and the use of pharmacologic agents to reduce the risk of pulmonary aspiration: application to healthy patients undergoing elective procedures: an updated report by the American Society of Anesthesiologists Task Force on preoperative fasting and the use of pharmacologic agents to reduce the risk of pulmonary aspiration. Anesthesiology 2017; 126(3):376–93.

13. Fleisher LA, Fleischmann KE, Auerbach AD, et al. 2014 ACC/AHA guideline on perioperative cardiovascular evaluation and management of patients undergoing noncardiac surgery: executive summary: a report of the American College of Cardiology/American Heart Association Task Force on practice guidelines. Developed in collaboration with the American College of Surgeons, American Society of Anesthesiologists, American Society of Echocardiography, American Society of Nuclear Cardiology, Heart Rhythm Society, Society for Cardiovascular Angiography and Interventions, Society of Cardiovascular Anesthesiologists, and Society of Vascular Medicine Endorsed by the Society of Hospital Medicine. J Nucl Cardiol 2015;22(1):162–215.

14. Narouze S, Benzon HT, Provenzano D, et al. Interventional spine and pain procedures in patients on antiplatelet and anticoagulant medications (second edition): guidelines from the American Society of Regional Anesthesia and Pain Medicine, the European Society of Regional Anaesthesia and Pain Therapy, the American Academy of Pain Medicine, the International Neuromodulation Society, the North American Neuromodulation Society, and the World Institute of Pain. Reg Anesth Pain Med 2018;43(3): 225–62.

15. Schlitzkus LL, Summers JI, Schenarts PJ. Rapid reversal of novel anticoagulant and antiplatelet medications in general surgery emergencies. Surg Clin North Am 2018;98(5):1073–80.

16. Maggard Gibbons M, Ulloa JG, Macqueen IT, et al. Management of antiplatelet therapy among patients on antiplatelet therapy for coronary or cerebrovascular disease or with prior percutaneous cardiac interventions undergoing elective surgery: a systematic review. VA ESP Project #5-226;2017.

17. O'Malley C, Cunningham AJ. Physiologic changes during laparoscopy. Anesthesiol Clin North America 2001;19(1):1–19.

18. Odeberg S, Ljungqvist O, Svenberg T, et al. Haemodynamic effects of pneumoperitoneum and the influence of posture during anaesthesia for laparoscopic surgery. Acta Anaesthesiol Scand 1994;38(3): 276–83.

19. Bartels K, Esper SA, Thiele RH. Blood pressure monitoring for the anesthesiologist: a practical review. Anesth Analg 2016;122(6):1866–79.

20. Thiele RH, Durieux ME. Arterial waveform analysis for the anesthesiologist: past, present, and future concepts. Anesth Analg 2011;113(4):766–76.

21. Han L, Su Y, Xiong H, et al. Oxycodone versus sufentanil in adult patient-controlled intravenous analgesia after abdominal surgery: a prospective, randomized, double-blinded, multiple-center clinical trial. Medicine (Baltimore) 2018;97(31):e11552.

22. Sultana A, Torres D, Schumann R. Special indications for opioid free anaesthesia and analgesia, patient and procedure related: including obesity, sleep apnoea, chronic obstructive pulmonary disease, complex regional pain syndromes, opioid addiction and cancer surgery. Best Pract Res Clin Anaesthesiol 2017;31(4):547–60.

23. de Boer HD, Detriche O, Forget P. Opioid-related side effects: postoperative ileus, urinary retention, nausea and vomiting, and shivering. A review of the literature. Best Pract Res Clin Anaesthesiol 2017;31(4):499–504.

24. Dotson K, Kiger J, Carpenter C, et al. Alignment of cricoid cartilage and esophagus and its potential influence on the effectiveness of Sellick maneuver in children. Pediatr Emerg Care 2010;26(10):722–5.

25. Landsman I. Cricoid pressure: indications and complications. Paediatr Anaesth 2004;14(1):43–7.

26. Algie CM, Mahar RK, Tan HB, et al. Effectiveness and risks of cricoid pressure during rapid sequence induction for endotracheal intubation. Cochrane Database Syst Rev 2015;(11):CD011656.

27. Michael Dunham C, Hileman BM, Hutchinson AE, et al. Evaluation of operating room reverse Trendelenburg positioning and its effect on postoperative hypoxemia, aspiration, and length of stay: a retrospective study of consecutive patients. Perioper Med (Lond) 2017;6:10. eCollection 2017.

28. Lohser J, Kulkarni V, Brodsky JB. Anesthesia for thoracic surgery in morbidly obese patients. Curr Opin Anaesthesiol 2007;20(1):10–4.

29. Koziol CA, Cuddeford JD, Moos DD. Assessing the force generated with application of cricoid pressure. AORN J 2000;72(6):1018–28, 1030.

30. Bauer C, Winter C, Hentz JG, et al. Bronchial blocker compared to double-lumen tube for one-lung ventilation during thoracoscopy. Acta Anaesthesiol Scand 2001;45(2):250–4.

31. Kosarek L, Busch E, Abbas A, et al. Effective use of bronchial blockers in lung isolation surgery: an analysis of 130 cases. Ochsner J 2013;13(3):389–93.

32. Joshi GP. Inhalational techniques in ambulatory anesthesia. Anesthesiol Clin North America 2003; 21(2):263–72.

33. Tonner PH, Scholz J. Total intravenous or balanced anaesthesia in ambulatory surgery? Curr Opin Anaesthesiol 2000;13(6):631–6.

34. Mikuni I, Harada S, Yakushiji R, et al. Effects of changing from sevoflurane to desflurane on the

recovery profile after sevoflurane induction: a randomized controlled study. Can J Anaesth 2016; 63(3):290–7.

35. Staehr-Rye AK, Rasmussen LS, Rosenberg J, et al. Surgical space conditions during low-pressure laparoscopic cholecystectomy with deep versus moderate neuromuscular blockade: a randomized clinical study. Anesth Analg 2014; 119(5):1084–92.

36. Carron M, Zarantonello F, Tellaroli P, et al. Efficacy and safety of sugammadex compared to neostigmine for reversal of neuromuscular blockade: a meta-analysis of randomized controlled trials. J Clin Anesth 2016;35:1–12.

37. Valenza F, Vagginelli F, Tiby A, et al. Effects of the beach chair position, positive end-expiratory pressure, and pneumoperitoneum on respiratory function in morbidly obese patients during anesthesia and paralysis. Anesthesiology 2007;107(5): 725–32.

38. Remistico PP, Araujo S, de Figueiredo LC, et al. Impact of alveolar recruitment maneuver in the postoperative period of videolaparoscopic bariatric surgery. Rev Bras Anestesiol 2011;61(2):163–8, 169-76, 88-94.

39. Pearse RM, Harrison DA, MacDonald N, et al. Effect of a perioperative, cardiac output-guided hemodynamic therapy algorithm on outcomes following major gastrointestinal surgery: a randomized clinical trial and systematic review. JAMA 2014;311(21): 2181–90.

40. Manning MW, Dunkman WJ, Miller TE. Perioperative fluid and hemodynamic management within an enhanced recovery pathway. J Surg Oncol 2017; 116(5):592–600.

41. Gupta R, Gan TJ. Peri-operative fluid management to enhance recovery. Anaesthesia 2016;71(Suppl 1):40–5.

42. Schauer PR, Meyers WC, Eubanks S, et al. Mechanisms of gastric and esophageal perforations during laparoscopic Nissen fundoplication. Ann Surg 1996; 223(1):43–52.

43. Novitsky YW, Kercher KW, Callery MP, et al. Is the use of a bougie necessary for laparoscopic Nissen fundoplication? Arch Surg 2002;137(4):402–6.

44. Jarral OA, Athanasiou T, Hanna GB, et al. Is an intra-oesophageal bougie of use during Nissen fundoplication? Interact Cardiovasc Thorac Surg 2012;14(6): 828–33.

45. Luketich JD, Nason KS, Christie NA, et al. Outcomes after a decade of laparoscopic giant paraesophageal hernia repair. J Thorac Cardiovasc Surg 2010; 139(2):395–404, 404.e1.

46. Lowham AS, Filipi CJ, Hinder RA, et al. Mechanisms and avoidance of esophageal perforation by anesthesia personnel during laparoscopic foregut surgery. Surg Endosc 1996;10(10):979–82.

47. Srivastava A, Niranjan A. Secrets of safe laparoscopic surgery: anaesthetic and surgical considerations. J Minim Access Surg 2010;6(4):91–4.

48. Wahba RW, Tessler MJ, Kleiman SJ. Acute ventilatory complications during laparoscopic upper abdominal surgery. Can J Anaesth 1996;43(1): 77–83.

49. Machairiotis N, Kougioumtzi I, Dryllis G, et al. Laparoscopy induced pneumothorax. J Thorac Dis 2014; 6(Suppl 4):S404–6.

50. Kockerling F, Schug-Pass C, Bittner R. A word of caution: never use tacks for mesh fixation to the diaphragm! Surg Endosc 2018;32(7):3295–302.

51. Stockhausen S, Kernbach-Wighton G, Madea B, et al. Rare causes of iatrogenic pericardial tamponade: 2 case reports. Arch Kriminol 2017;239(1–2): 36–44.

52. McClellan JM, Nelson D, Martin M. Hemopericardium after laparoscopic perihiatal procedures: high index of suspicion facilitates early diagnosis and successful nonoperative management. Surg Obes Relat Dis 2016;12(3):e27–31.

53. Porter JM. Diagnostic laparoscopy and laparoscopic transdiaphragmatic pericardial window in a patient with an epigastric stab wound: a case report. J Laparoendosc Surg 1996;6(1):51–4.

54. Mann GB, Nguyen H, Corbet J. Laparoscopic creation of pericardial window. Aust N Z J Surg 1994; 64(12):853–5.

55. Schmandra TC, Mierdl S, Bauer H, et al. Transoesophageal echocardiography shows high risk of gas embolism during laparoscopic hepatic resection under carbon dioxide pneumoperitoneum. Br J Surg 2002;89(7):870–6.

56. Pruszczyk P, Torbicki A, Pacho R, et al. Noninvasive diagnosis of suspected severe pulmonary embolism: transesophageal echocardiography vs spiral CT. Chest 1997;112(3):722–8.

57. Desciak MC, Martin DE. Perioperative pulmonary embolism: diagnosis and anesthetic management. J Clin Anesth 2011;23(2):153–65.

58. Vijayaraghavan N, Sistla SC, Kundra P, et al. Comparison of standard-pressure and low-pressure pneumoperitoneum in laparoscopic cholecystectomy: a double blinded randomized controlled study. Surg Laparosc Endosc Percutan Tech 2014; 24(2):127–33.

59. Hua J, Gong J, Yao L, et al. Low-pressure versus standard-pressure pneumoperitoneum for laparoscopic cholecystectomy: a systematic review and meta-analysis. Am J Surg 2014;208(1): 143–50.

60. Helander EM, Webb MP, Bias M, et al. Use of regional anesthesia techniques: analysis of institutional enhanced recovery after surgery protocols for colorectal surgery. J Laparoendosc Adv Surg Tech A 2017;27(9):898–902.

61. Pirrera B, Alagna V, Lucchi A, et al. Transversus abdominis plane (TAP) block versus thoracic epidural analgesia (TEA) in laparoscopic colon surgery in the ERAS program. Surg Endosc 2018;32(1): 376–82.

62. Vyas KS, Rajendran S, Morrison SD, et al. Systematic review of liposomal bupivacaine (exparel) for postoperative analgesia. Plast Reconstr Surg 2016; 138(4):748e-56e.

63. Ong CK, Seymour RA, Lirk P, et al. Combining paracetamol (acetaminophen) with nonsteroidal antiinflammatory drugs: a qualitative systematic review of analgesic efficacy for acute postoperative pain. Anesth Analg 2010;110(4):1170–9.

64. Gupta A, Bah M. NSAIDs in the treatment of postoperative pain. Curr Pain Headache Rep 2016; 20(11):62.

65. Molina JC, Misariu AM, Nicolau I, et al. Same day discharge for benign laparoscopic hiatal surgery: a feasibility analysis. Surg Endosc 2018;32(2): 937–44.

66. Levy BF, Scott MJ, Fawcett WJ, et al. Optimizing patient outcomes in laparoscopic surgery. Colorectal Dis 2011;13(Suppl 7):8–11.

UNITED STATES POSTAL SERVICE®

Statement of Ownership, Management, and Circulation (All Periodicals Publications Except Requester Publications)

1. Publication Title	2. Publication Number	3. Filing Date
THORACIC SURGERY CLINICS	013 – 126	9/18/2019

4. Issue Frequency	5. Number of Issues Published Annually	6. Annual Subscription Price
FEB, MAY, AUG, NOV	4	$382.00

7. Complete Mailing Address of Known Office of Publication (Not printer) (Street, city, county, state, and ZIP+4®)

ELSEVIER INC.
230 Park Avenue, Suite 800
New York, NY 10169

Contact Person
STEPHEN R. BUSHING

Telephone (Include area code)
215-239-3688

8. Complete Mailing Address of Headquarters or General Business Office of Publisher (Not printer)

ELSEVIER INC.
230 Park Avenue, Suite 800
New York, NY 10169

9. Full Names and Complete Mailing Addresses of Publisher, Editor, and Managing Editor (Do not leave blank)

Publisher (Name and complete mailing address)

TAYLOR BALL, ELSEVIER INC.
1600 JOHN F KENNEDY BLVD. SUITE 1800
PHILADELPHIA, PA 19103-2899

Editor (Name and complete mailing address)

JOHN VASSALLO, ELSEVIER INC.
1600 JOHN F KENNEDY BLVD. SUITE 1800
PHILADELPHIA, PA 19103-2899

Managing Editor (Name and complete mailing address)

PATRICK MANLEY, ELSEVIER INC.
1600 JOHN F KENNEDY BLVD. SUITE 1800
PHILADELPHIA, PA 19103-2899

10. Owner (Do not leave blank. If the publication is owned by a corporation, give the name and address of the corporation immediately followed by the names and addresses of all stockholders owning or holding 1 percent or more of the total amount of stock. If not owned by a corporation, give the names and addresses of the individual owners. If owned by a partnership or other unincorporated firm, give its name and address as well as those of each individual owner. If the publication is published by a nonprofit organization, give its name and address.)

Full Name	Complete Mailing Address
WHOLLY OWNED SUBSIDIARY OF REED/ELSEVIER, US HOLDINGS	1600 JOHN F KENNEDY BLVD. SUITE 1800 PHILADELPHIA, PA 19103-2899

11. Known Bondholders, Mortgagees, and Other Security Holders Owning or Holding 1 Percent or More of Total Amount of Bonds, Mortgages, or Other Securities. If none, check box ▶ ☐ None

Full Name	Complete Mailing Address
N/A	

12. Tax Status (For completion by nonprofit organizations authorized to mail at nonprofit rates) (Check one)
The purpose, function, and nonprofit status of this organization and the exempt status for federal income tax purposes:
☒ Has Not Changed During Preceding 12 Months
☐ Has Changed During Preceding 12 Months (Publisher must submit explanation of change with this statement)

PS Form 3526, July 2014 [Page 1 of 4 (see instructions page 4)]   PSN: 7530-01-000-9931   PRIVACY NOTICE: See our privacy policy on www.usps.com.

13. Publication Title	14. Issue Date for Circulation Data Below
THORACIC SURGERY CLINICS	AUGUST 2019

15. Extent and Nature of Circulation		Average No. Copies Each Issue During Preceding 12 Months	No. Copies of Single Issue Published Nearest to Filing Date
a. Total Number of Copies (Net press run)		217	238
b. Paid Circulation (By Mail and Outside the Mail)	(1) Mailed Outside-County Paid Subscriptions Stated on PS Form 3541 (Include paid distribution above nominal rate, advertiser's proof copies, and exchange copies)	87	80
	(2) Mailed In-County Paid Subscriptions Stated on PS Form 3541 (Include paid distribution above nominal rate, advertiser's proof copies, and exchange copies)	0	0
	(3) Paid Distribution Outside the Mails Including Sales Through Dealers and Carriers, Street Vendors, Counter Sales, and Other Paid Distribution Outside USPS®	73	65
	(4) Paid Distribution by Other Classes of Mail Through the USPS (e.g. First-Class Mail®)	0	0
c. Total Paid Distribution (Sum of 15b (1), (2), (3), and (4))	▶	160	145
d. Free or Nominal Rate Distribution (By Mail and Outside the Mail)	(1) Free or Nominal Rate Outside-County Copies included on PS Form 3541	42	68
	(2) Free or Nominal Rate In-County Copies Included on PS Form 3541	0	0
	(3) Free or Nominal Rate Copies Mailed at Other Classes Through the USPS (e.g. First-Class Mail)	0	0
	(4) Free or Nominal Rate Distribution Outside the Mail (Carriers or other means)	0	0
e. Total Free or Nominal Rate Distribution (Sum of 15d (1), (2), (3) and (4))	▶	42	68
f. Total Distribution (Sum of 15c and 15e)	▶	202	213
g. Copies not Distributed (See Instructions to Publishers #4 (page #3))	▶	15	25
h. Total (Sum of 15f and g)	▶	217	238
i. Percent Paid (15c divided by 15f times 100)	▶	79.1%	68.08%

* If you are claiming electronic copies, go to line 16 on page 3. If you are not claiming electronic copies, skip to line 17 on page 3.

16. Electronic Copy Circulation		Average No. Copies Each Issue During Preceding 12 Months	No. Copies of Single Issue Published Nearest to Filing Date
a. Paid Electronic Copies	▶		
b. Total Paid Print Copies (Line 15c) + Paid Electronic Copies (Line 16a)	▶		
c. Total Print Distribution (Line 15f) + Paid Electronic Copies (Line 16a)	▶		
d. Percent Paid (Both Print & Electronic Copies) (16b divided by 16c × 100)	▶		

☒ I certify that 50% of all my distributed copies (electronic and print) are paid above a nominal price.

17. Publication of Statement of Ownership

☒ If the publication is a general publication, publication of this statement is required. Will be printed in the NOVEMBER 2019 issue of this publication.   ☐ Publication not required.

18. Signature and Title of Editor, Publisher, Business Manager, or Owner

[signature] Stephen R. Bushing   Date 9/18/2019

STEPHEN R. BUSHING - INVENTORY DISTRIBUTION CONTROL MANAGER

I certify that all information furnished on this form is true and complete. I understand that anyone who furnishes false or misleading information on this form or who omits material or information requested on the form may be subject to criminal sanctions (including fines and imprisonment) and/or civil sanctions (including civil penalties).

PS Form 3526, July 2014 (Page 3 of 4)   PRIVACY NOTICE: See our privacy policy on www.usps.com.

Printed and bound by CPI Group (UK) Ltd, Croydon, CR0 4YY

08/05/2025

01864747-0008